The Great Break

DATE			

The Great Break
A Short History of the Separation of Medical Science from Religion

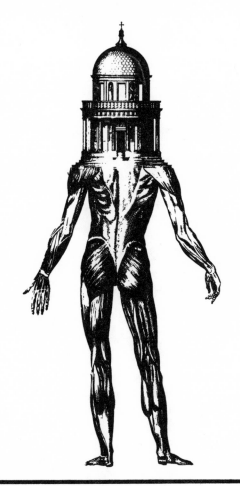

Joseph Mauceri, M.D.

P·U·L·S·E

SOCIAL SCIENCE & HISTORY DIVISION
EDUCATION & PHILOSOPHY SECTION

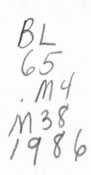

Published by P·U·L·S·E Books, a division of Station Hill Press, Inc., Barrytown, NY 12507.

Produced by the Institute for Publishing Arts, Barrytown, NY 12507, a not-for-profit, tax-exempt organization.

Designed by Susan Quasha.

Library of Congress Cataloging-in-Publication Data

Mauceri, Joseph, 1943–
  The great break.

  Bibliography: p.
  Includes index.
  1. Medicine—Religious aspects—History. 2. Religion
and science—History. I. Title. [DNLM: 1. Religion
and Medicine—history. WZ 40 M447g]
  BL65.M4M38 1986   610'.9   86-8702
  ISBN 0-940170-13-2

$$592\ 27764$$

Manufactured in the United States of America.

for my mother
who always rescued the truth

Contents

Introduction

The age of science was announced in a political letter. In 1902 the infamous Germanophile Houston Chamberlain wrote to Kaiser Wilhelm; "We have arrived at a turning point in history. . .the new world is the world of science and it is science which will dominate."[1] Chamberlain had a specific idea in mind, the idea of a "War Civilization," as Wagner said, but the truth of Chamberlain's vision would penetrate every area of modern life. Twentieth century man was ready for the message, ready for the change. It would be a great turning point indeed. Nothing has gripped modern man so powerfully, so completely, even daring him to proclaim himself free of the old hobgoblins, philosophy and religion. There may have been a time when these made sense but that was because nothing else did. Now we have knowledge, science, the hangman of superstition.

Hegel once wrote that, "Knowledge has taken possession of all material and given it the necessary connection."[2] Hegel realized that science was already a persuasive instrument, an instrument which man would have to reckon with, but Hegel also knew that scientific knowledge was "still unable to give the absolute connection." Modern man, however, has lost sight of the absolute connection and is satisfied with the necessary connection. He is not interested in any other because scientific triumphs are an immediate and unimpeachable witness to the power of positive knowledge. Why should men who have tamed the atom and struck at the core of life be concerned with the "Absolute connection?" Thus, with deceptive ease they have embraced science and no longer seek anything else. They are very clear about all of this; they can tell you precisely what they believe; progress, technology, the control of nature, scientific sociology, rationalism. They will sit with you with arms folded, feet up, and speak of all of this right in the middle of the last part of the most calamitous century in history, forgetting that all of those have been tools for the absolute debasement of men in our time. The only real fear, they will say, was the fear of God, an idea derived from fear born of ignorance and then used to instill both. It was all a misunderstanding . . . we confused an infantile hope (God exists) with a previously unthinkable reality (what if God is not?).

There is deep irony here for the scientific age is heir to a heritage which runs deep in our civilization, a heritage rooted in the principles of rational creation and natural law. Modern man, however, has let go of these because of their unpleasant theological odor and fastened on to the promise of science the way he once bowed in reverence. Ortgega said it well, we are always in the grip of a belief.

What is this new belief? It is an intellectual Procrustes which aims to define the origins of cosmos and life, the basis for man's social arrangements and political life, even the meaning of his existence. The new religion, science, promised us unlimited power, and we eagerly placed our collective psyche in conformity with the promise. But scientific power has not been bought cheaply, somewhere along the way we lost sight of another truth, one that C. S. Lewis grasped when he said, "Man's power over nature turns out to be power executed by some men over other men with nature as its instrument."[3] The scientist still dreams of power while he misses the awful irony. He is awed by his science but fears all of the genies it loosens. Look at the splicing of the gene and the splitting of the atom. Not a day goes by without reference to the bomb or to the potential horror in the experimental creation of life forms. The bomb, after all, is the power of annihilation, and DNA is the "proof" that man is only molecular. Yet each new scientific advance begins to take on a life of its own so that technical miracles soon become life-like extensions of the human personality and the distinction between the man and the machine blurs. Then man becomes the slave of utility. We are told that science is morally neutral and that man is still in charge, but when the indifferent machine is in the hands of an indifferent mechanic . . . well, the terrible thing has already happened and "modern man is placed in a condition of perplexity by confusing the knowledge he can prove with the conviction by which he lives."[4]

There was a time when man was not in possession of controlling knowledge yet he did not feel an absence of control. He felt his place in the cosmic order, and over the centuries used his reason to begin to explicate that order. With the eye of reason, the scientific method, man looked again to "know" the cosmos because he already believed in its rationality. At the end of the Renaissance, after a hiatus spent contemplating theology and philosophy, man began the enterprise of making science in earnest, but it was an enterprise conducted within a theological universe. Thus, as great names in the story passed, their new knowledge did not raise new doubts. Men still labored with a sense of awe, exhilarating in the discovery that, "The most incomprehensible thing about the universe (is) its comprehensibility."[5] Copernicus saw his work as the explication of the "Great Artificer," and Kepler and Newton believed that their laws fit well the plan of ordered creation. Cesalpinus and Harvey, the physicians, saw this grand plan in the harmony and perfection of the movement of the life principle. Leeuwenhoek and Schwammerdam magnified "morbid" matter and discovered "animalcules," tiny life. Everywhere man looked, order prevailed. Finally, so it seemed, even the twentieth century atom of orbiting electrons (planets) and central neutrons (suns) extended the harmonious whole to the extremes of the cosmic scale.

Science validated the order of nature, but it also imposed its will on her processes, so that the order became less important as the power grew. Then the great mistake took hold, the idea of science was installed over and above life and meaning. Knowledge became the absolute connection and was changed so that all which was not provable with the eye of reason was rejected. Now only the verifiable is "real." This idea has overtaken all intellectual life and has pushed reason to the extreme so that only those questions which are lexically consistent with the "verification principle" may be asked. A question must be in principle capable of being answered by an empirical test or else it is nonsense. Spiritual questions and questions of "existential" meaning are not only unanswerable, they are illogical. But even this scientific logic is strained by a rigorous rationalism which suggests the lexical arrangement is also insufficient to the truth. That must be left to a mathematical-logical philosophy untainted by the possibilities of falsification inherent in traditional science and our ordinary way of speaking and thinking. This "philosophy" can only collapse in nihilism, and nihilism, of course, is the other side of rationalism: nihilism speaks eloquently the intellectual poverty of the apotheosis of reason.

The story of this growth of science to its place in modern life, any story of the history of scientific progress, cannot be told without tracing the evolution of medical thought. Certainly medicine is more intimately linked to the life and culture of man than the other sciences because of its special vigilance against death and its preoccupation with the care of the sick man. Thus, throughout history, medical thought has paralleled and often anticipated the growth of natural philosophy. Indeed, it could be fairly said that medicine is the first science because of its special place in the business of communities of men, back to the oldest; even ancient medicine had to be sufficiently successful as a practical art, it had to help often enough that it could help again, and that was the first step in putting medicine on a scientific footing. But there is another reason for medicine's special place in our story. Very early medicine and religion were closey linked because birth, death, illness and cure were mysterious events with spiritual and cosmic meaning. Medicine still had to be more than a methodology, it had to see man in all of his existential precariousness. It had to keep the religious and philosophical in view so that their truths would satisfy when medicine could no longer bring a cure. The physician ministered to his patient, "to sometimes cure, often to help, always console,"[6] because he shared in his patient's experience by sharing in its meaning. As medical thought matured and became more scientific it still made theological sense, if in a different way, by showing that disease is not necessarily the curse of an invisible hand but is in the natural order of things, a view consistent with Western Judeo-Christian thought.

The present situation represents a radical break for science and medicine from their common past. Medicine is now, unhappily, obsessively factual so that it cannot allow any place for the philosophical or the spiritual. In the physical and chemical sciences which inform medical theory this is of no real danger, but in the art of medicine this goes to the very heart of the mission. But there is a theoretical hazard as well; when scientific medicine offers strictly materialistic theories of life and consciousness it stands man on his head. In this regard, of course, scientific medicine has lost its connection with previous thought which acknowledged that man and his world issued from Intelligence and Rational Creation, for in the climate of thought which once prevailed, medicine and science made sense because they could only have developed in a world which made sense. The Western scientific experience served the idea of a "Scientific God," a God who laid out His world like a good city planner, "Demiurgos." In other places, for other civilizations, God was less a city planner and more a whimsical God of urban sprawl; if He were in the construction business it would have been Hong Kong, the chaos of a God detached from his Creation. This has been the Eastern view, a world and cosmos of ceaseless flux in which the rationality of creation is denied because of desire to flee the pain of living it. This was one reason why science was as impossible in the East as it has been compelling in the West.

The Hindu cosmological view, for instance, had little "cosmos" and lots of "view," a long metaphysical view wrapped in pessimism and set on a psychological meeting of consciousness with the universe beyond time and place. The Hindu man was satisfied with his philosophy so he relaxed his efforts in science even though he made some advances in astronomy, geometry and medicinal cures. It was the same in China, Egypt and Chaldea, and at a different times during the Greek period. There was no overwhelming necessity to develop natural science for its own sake because the cosmological problem had been "answered." Western man, however, intensified efforts in the natural and physical sciences, not so much to establish the scientific as the explanation as by way of discovering that it verified his intuition. Science was supposed to make man more at home in his reality.

Scientific achievement and its related technological successes, however, brought a new and thoroughly modern form of doubt. Obviously, no one man, no single event or historical period marks the shift. The displacement of the old emphasis by the new knowledge was a slow process and biology and medicine, as they incorporated the reductionist methods, played an important part in bringing the scientific world view into the main stream of modern culture. Enlightenment philosophy defined the issue; reason can stand on its own, it can throw away the theological crutches. The scientific, industrial age added another idol, the machine, which soon separated man from his previously personal relation to the rhythm and pulse of nature and work. This depersonalization did not necessarily lessen human drudgery but it did prepare man for the complete mechanization of life in the twentieth century. Nineteenth century physics, biology and medicine took this psychological preparation much further. The laboratory isolated the forces of nature and the vital functions of life and demystified them. This was accomplished in two ways. Laboratory science gave names to processes and then measured their effects. Like his primitive forebears who named the cosmic forces and made a reckoning of their "function" into a nature religion, the scientist named the functions and described causality, creating a knowledge religion. Intoxicated by his new power, the scientist lost interest in the quest for meaning. In his exulting over finding out how it is, he no longer asked why it is. It only mattered to him that this new religion, science, is about power... power works!

Medicine, once again, shows itself to be a special case. Biology and medicine, after all, are "life" sciences but no matter how much scientists probe and test in the laboratory, the mysteries of life elude them. Oh, the scientists can describe mechanisms and processes and tell us "how" it is, how life and consciousness are molecular or biochemical, e.g., but these descriptions are not explanations, and certainly tell us nothing about why there is life, and why it is as it is for each of us uniquely. Biomedical research has certainly striven in earnest to answer the question why things are as they are, but the returns have only further deepened the surrounding darkness. Contemporary scientific medicine, however, has taken the accumulated knowledge of the laboratory to mean that all life, including human life, is a function of matter. This formulation even conforms very well to the evolutionary one. Living things are in their essence material things, and the highest order of living things, man, takes his origins from the lowest. The most telling part of this scientific philosophy is the connection scientists now make between the living and the inanimate. Life, itself, has its origins in primordial matter.

This materialism has placed medicine in philosophical, practical and ethical difficulties. The philosophical problem derives from the medical model: illness and disease, somatic and psychic, are functions of perturbations in a material body. Thus medicine which should be the science par excellence of the whole man violates its own ideal by accepting the scientific dismissal of spirit. The practical problem is derivative. The physician must be scientific, he must objectify the problem of the sick man and make it a clinical problem. This excludes all evidence that is not quantifiable and cannot be incorporated into some abstract collection of data. On the other hand, every doctor who has ever thought about the sick man knows that disease is far more shadowy than that. Whatever it is that stalks the sick man it is no mere germ or bug or only some physiologic disturbance. Disease grips the whole man just as the whole man, psyche and soma, grapples with the disease. The entire plot is played out mysteriously and uniquely each time the patient meets his disease, and for the physician at the bedside objectivity may be a "necessary" connection but it is hardly the "absolute" one.

The ethical problem is related to the others. The cold objectification demanded by the scientific mind removes it from the ethical by its own claim that it cannot be value oriented. That would only be an impediment to the specific mission at hand, and to the progress of science in general. The unhappy result in medicine is that doctors are so unsure of their mission that others are now called to the bedside; ethicists, philosophers and leglists. In a scientific age where every man is a "specialist," ethical or moral questions are weighed like any other diagnostic problem while the doctor stands by with his arms folded. And this applies equally to the whole question of the limits of medical technology, a question which touches the human being from conception to the moment he draws his last breath in the highly mechanized environ which characterizes modern medicine. If medical ethics rests on contemporary scientific philosophy, then the notion of functional matter allows everything, everything from gene manipulations to technically managed death.

The truth of Chamberlain's dictum, then, is obvious everywhere we turn today. Few would question the importance of man's scientific efforts and the need to continue. Science counts, it is part of the human epic and its successes have raised our material condition to an extraordinary level. But this hardly allows that science can define human life and consciousness and the meaning of life on its own terms. These are questions whose answers reside in the philosophical and theological realm, they are not question that we can assault in a laboratory. Science only adds to the mystery by adding to the incalculable number of phenomena, their order, and their complexity. Certainly the atom and the DNA particle are not the last advances science will make, they have only heightened the questions. The primitive stuff of molecular biology can be cut or mixed as you like, it will not explain man, and elementary particles will not bridge matter and consciousness; relationships are not identities!

The questions the scientific age raises are not really new questions, they are the oldest questions in the long history of human thought. The first man who gazed into the heavens and the first shaman to call down the spirits on behalf of the sick man were not scientific, clearly, but they were hardly indifferent to the questions and that is why they did exactly what the evidence says they did. Only recently has that changed so it now seems that science has vanquished all other knowledge and established itself as the final arbiter of truth with a resulting antagonism between science and philosophical-religious inquiry which is the subject of our story, a story I have chosen to tell against the backdrop of the rise of scientific medicine because of my view that medicine is the oldest and most unique science.

As we begin I must remind you that a book is a lot like science; a description, not an explanation. Writers obscure the continuity of ideas and principles which motivated their subjects and they presume to mark off ages and periods as if they had a real existence while citing some men when many others made their contributions. That doesn't mean we should give up on the story, but we shouldn't forget the hazards in telling it. Accordingly, I proceed with all of the usual abuses.

The Great Break

The Shaman

Wonder, fear, exhilaration filled the mind of early man intellectually disarmed in his world. Overwhelmed by the power and unpredictability of natural forces he did what we can only say was the necessary thing, he deified the cosmic order. Primitive man sought a relation to it uninhibited by rational explanation. He viewed his world animistically and attached himself directly to its objects by a process of being in the things themselves. The heavens, living things and natural events or objects of immediate concern were personalized. There was an intimacy with storms and sunrises, stars and planets, animals and forests, birth and death. In a leap over the rational, he knew through his imagination, "grasping the truth" as Bachofen says, "at one stroke without intermediary levels."[1] Barfield would call it "original participation."[2] Man explained and developed meaning mythopoeically, not as the fabulous but as the real. Primal myths, creation myths and the mythologies of cosmic events disclosed a truth otherwise hidden by an rational encounter with them.

Such is one formulation of the way we moderns think it was at a time about which nothing is certain. It accepts the reality of animistic and mythopoetic thinking and sees man as a religious being. A second formulation recognizes such thinking in early man only to discredit him. He is simply irrational, imprisoned by fears. Man's mythmaking, his totems, his taboos, his gods were the nonsense products of an undeveloped intellect. There could be no meaning because man was yet incapable of thought. Meaning would have to wait for knowledge commensurate with man's use of his reason; it would have to wait for science. A third formulation is not unlike the first and can even accomodate the second. According to this view man is religious, not because he is in awe and ignorance of his world, but because he has fallen from a blessed state and can only restore meaning through another "irrational" leap. He must think another form of madness. He must violate the reality of the rational to achieve the truth of existence. This formulation has its genesis in revelation and its fulfillment in time and though this historical consciousness describes the ontological reality of time, the madness of this leap of faith lifts consciousness back into timelessness.

I think it is more than curious that the first formulation, which must keep to the evidence, discovers the religious in man. Early man, when he first sought meaning, sought it supernaturally. Nowhere is it written or does legend have it that man was to be born one day and for the rest of his life be blindly conducted to annihilation. Rather the creation myths and the urge to immortality gave meaning to being and made life something other than an absurdity of mere physical life. Medicine, in its rude beginnings, shared in this view and regard for the spiritual, as it did through most of its history, rarely separating its mission from a sense of higher meaning. So it is that the first healer we meet is a singular character, striking us both with the simplicity of his science and the profundity of his belief.

The outstanding figure of ancient medicine was the shaman, the mediator between the cosmic forces and the sick man, whose preeminence was an extension of the primitives' relation to the cosmos. The shaman approached the familiar and immediate aspects of natural phenomena with empirical consistency while he dealt with the esoteric or unpredictable aspects of nature on a magico-religious level. His role was a special one because he labored in a world of supernatural cause and effect, his methods a reflection of the primitive mind's grasp of reality which was decidedly intuitive and spiritual, transcendental and naturalistic. Primitives assigned personal and vital attributes to material reality so that behind or, more correctly, within each aspect of natural phenomena there was the informing principle of spirit which could have been a departed tribal figure, an ancestor, one of the gods or great spirits, the spirit of a totem animal or the deified elements of nature, the sun and the moon being the most obvious.

The primitive had a sense of the transcendant nature of time and reality, a sense characteristic of a great part of the world's archaic religions. The primitive man believed in a reality beyond both his own physical existence and the immediacy of things around him. The abode of the great spirit was beyond the physical world and unmeasurable in time, and there was the expectation that at death one would pass into this timelessness. Another aspect of primitive spirituality was the belief in the supernatural origins of the cosmos. Creation myths and myths of immortality, not only as life after death but as timelessness reaching back before individual existence, are found throughout the world. The primitive, of course, did not theorize or philosophize about all of this. He was neither the existentialist of his own condition nor the physicist of the cosmic reality. He simply believed.

The mysteriousness and spirituality of primitive belief meant that magic and religion were realities implied in the conduct of their daily living. Magic was employed to assist natural events while serving the totality of these events both in their physical and mystical aspect. This underscores both the practical and the spiritual aims of the magical rite. It was not an irrational exercise but one with internal consistency; the magical subserved the spiritual, ie., the unseen, transcendent forces that govern the universe and natural or cosmic events that affect man. The magical rite is a concession to the unseen, not as a rite of propitiation so much as a rite practically directed to a desired outcome. Magic is not mythology, and it does not by its accomplishment explicate any of the secrets of the unseen. Magic, rather, is witness to beliefs that the primitive mythologies already express. The great myths serve as the "exegesis of the symbols" of the primitive culture and provide the cosmological basis for primitive life. This is the religious sense that looms so large in primitive existence. Reality was indivisible and non-material, a spiritual wholeness that pervaded all elements of existence. The primitive lived as one with this natural order of the spirit.

The primitive had need of a specialist who might mediate between him and his reality. Each member of the tribe had possession of the common tribal heritage passed on by the spoken word as myth and symbolized in the totems and the prescribed totemic acts. The mediating function was not required for understanding these myths, symbols and prescriptions, but for satisfying them. The mediating man in illness and death, the shaman, was called upon because of his special ways of reaching the abode of the spirits, relations with whom determined health or sickness, fortune or calamity for the tribesman. The shaman's contact with the spiritual, therefore, had a practical utility, to heal. The shaman did this by bringing the sick man and the tribe into relation with the spirits through his invocations. The shaman's role was a dual role, he was a priest-healer, his spiritual passkey served his priestly role and at the same time this was used to assist him in his medical role. It is important to note, however, that the primitive did not impute the cure to the shaman's medicine but saw the cure working through his mediation. It was not his practical skill, though he possessed a good deal of that, but his transcendant skills, akin to the prophet's as a "specialist in ecstasy" that earned the shaman his status. His role was in keeping with the original sense of prophet, one to whom God has spoken a message to carry back, thus his "ex-stasis," his going out-of-himself, to mediate. The shaman was a special man, then, because the spiritual reality which he mediated and his art of healing could not be separated. He was preeminent because, in Eliade's phrase "at the archaic level of culture being is fused with the holy."[3]

Few of us are unfamiliar with the shaman's ways. They represent the very oldest rituals man has ever performed and they persist to this day in those ever shrinking parts of the world where man still lives in the primitive mode. Picture the shaman aside the sick man, adorned in the high fashion of his tribe, the exotic skins, the teeth and bones of animals, holding his amulets and charms, and his healing stick and fire. He had come upon the sick man to discover the lengthy history of the disease. The emphasis in that history was far removed from the modern doctor's interview for his questions probed not for symptoms but for the spiritual fault in the victim. Had the sick man, for instance, violated a tribal taboo: Had he killed a totem animal? Had he transgressed or violated nature, harmed a kinsman or an animal without need? Had he displeased the great spirit? And if the shaman hears an answer, then he can begin to work through the knowledge it brings. He will summon all of his technical apparatus, his drums, his fire, his totem symbols, to begin his mystical ascent to the great spirits to find the cure. His chant, his dance trance and his "delirium" are an integral part of this. They are his way of making his ascent, of reaching the plane of mediation. He can flee the sensible world to the spiritual and return carrying the cure. He will speak those words he heard on his journey into the ear of the sick man, for he carries in his own psyche the expectation of the sick one and the promise of healing.

The shaman carries the expectation of the community as well, for by his ecstacy he is able to mediate for the community. When the parched earth gives up its "dust spirit" to the "great wind" the shaman will speak for the rains to come. When the waters flood, he will dance for the sunrise to come, and when the sick one dies he will call the ancestors and the great spirit to take the departed safely and he will speak, even if silently, the hope of all in his tribe. He is the preeminent mediating one because "he is expert in remedying the precariousness and impurity of human existence."[4] We, conditioned to the promise of validation through science, must remain quiet before all of this. It is incorrect to call the primitive prelogical and his conduct irrational. What we see is belief and we can only be silent in its presence.

The shaman is the logical, indeed the only possible choice as mediator in the primitive world for if the sick one suffered because of a violation or taboo or any offense against the spirits then his illness is a dysfunction of the soul, and a cure can only be found in the spiritual domain. The American Indian, for instance, was governed by the mystical view of life and concordant genesis and after-life myths. The Indian's world was also populated by spirits and disease had mystical meaning. The sick man might be taken ill by the ghost of an animal he had mistreated or by the spirit of an ancestor he dishonored. The sick man may have shown a disregard for nature or had an unfulfilled dream wish. He may have been a coward in battle, fainthearted on the hunt or cruel to the weak. The medicine man, in any case, would consult the sick man as to the circumstances. Then he would undertake his ritual magic, call forth the spirit of the dead animal or propitiate the nature spirits. If the sick one had been hexed, the shaman would pray over him to undo the malevolent effects of the hex. The Indian, like the primitive, was non-literate and the lack of the written word made him over-committed to the spoken word which was a powerful force in the healing. When the shaman spoke into the ear of the sick man it was only by what he spoke, that he spoke at all, that a cure could come.

The shaman was not without technical skills, however, as he could not long have maintained a preeminent character in the face of recurring failure. Those skills are obscured by time but sufficient observation of contemporary primitives and Native American Indians, about whose healing much has been written by explorers and priests, assure us that shamanistic practices were often technically valid and had an empirical basis. The shaman's task, remember, was specific, he was engaged to make the sick well.

The primitive healer was an expert in herbal remedies, poison therapy, ritual bathing, massage, a crude iatro-chemistry, concoction and decoction, music and verbal therapy. He was versed in the extensive pharmacoepia of herbals and familiar with other remedies and methods. Indians had, for example, anethesia from cocoa leaves and methyl salicylate from sweet birch, emetics such as epecac, cathartics like cascara and podophyllin from the may apple root, and worm medicine from pink root. Alum root was applied to wounds and ulcers as a styptic, cranberry was used as a diuretic and many bark and leaf decoctions employed against fever, ague and pain. Garlic and onions, with alium, were used as antibacterials and digestives, Ginseng for rheumatism and rejuvenation of the sex faculties and slowing of the aging process. The shaman had primitive surgical knowhow as well. The medicine man could repair fractures, cauterize wounds and assist birthing with mechanical and obstetrical devices. He also used a method of skullsurgery (trephining) practiced since the very earliest days. This widespread and ancient practice is of uncertain purpose or origin. It might well have been a method of treating the many brain hemorrhages and injuries caused by primitive weapons, clubs and stones. The trephine procedure was employed in these cases to relieve pressure much as a craniotomy is performed today. Then again, the trephining may have been a magical rite to relieve the possessed man of his demons, opening the skull so that the frenzy or madness would go elsewhere, as devils into swine.

The Indians were in possession of rudimentary contraceptive herbs and apparently knew the benefit of suckling as their children were often spaced several years apart. They also knew the menstrual cycle and its relationship to fertility. Delivery itself was accomplished with a minimum of discomfort and the placenta was always expelled by appropriate external massage, a method only later practiced in Europe. The treatment of wounds and burns with herbals and chemical mixtures was commonly applied, both for pain relief and infection control. Puff balls and spider webs were used as antihemorrhagics and tourniquets were employed to close down the vessels or reduce the flow of venom in the snake bite.

All of these remedies and practices had experiential validity, they represent primitive empirical science. Success, however often interrupted by failure, could bring a particular remedy or technique to regular application even though the theory or principle behind its application and efficacy would not be sought. Yet some sense of cause and effect must have been followed as particular herbs, for instance, were applied for specific cases and withheld in others. The magical arts and rites were employed to assist the herbs and were employed as the primary mode when an illness appeared without any specific herbal remedy being available to deal with it. The magic in either situation persisted because, as Malinowski noted, "in human memory the testimony of a positive case always overshadows the negative one."[5] If, in the trance dance, the healing chant or word therapy were occasionally effective, their efficacy was confirmed. The shaman endured not because he labored in ignorance but because his presence added something to nature, while in the service of nature he seemed able to call forth more from it. He joined his empirical skill to his magical knowledge to satisfy the entire realm of being. But the magical was bound to the religious so that the sacred and the profane converged in the same man because the supernatural and the natural converged in disease and death. The medicine man of North America, even today, is not unlike the shaman of old.

The convergence of the sacred and the profane made the primitive particularly sensitive to the care of nature and the conservation of its resources. Animal life was respected and the purity of water, air and forest was a part of Indian life, even if for theological rather than medical reasons. On the other hand, the Indians saw the great value in the preservation of all of this for health. It was their world, they would tend it with care.

There is another aspect of primitive and Indian life that is hardly inconsequential for us, aside from the medical and healing practices. Malinowski notes that the real point of animism for these peoples was the desire for the afterlife, a state anticipated in their various cosmogenic myths. Myths, remember, are a retelling of the first mysteries of life and a revelation about the cosmic forces. Eliade comments that "myth could only be grasped insofar as it revealed something as having been fully manifested and created and exemplary since it was the foundation of a structure of reality as well as a kind of human behavior."[6] By being exemplary it described the universal condition and the origin of community. By being religious it answered the question of the nature of existence and being, contained the archetypes for belief, and revealed the way to immortality.

All civilization which followed upon primitive society have had to satisfy similar religious requirements. Hindu, the Chinese, the Egyptian, Babylonian, Chaldean, Persian and early Greek civilizations had cosmogenic and primal myths virtually identical in their elaboration of basic truths. Significantly, the first "sciences" in all of these civilizations were astronomy and healing and the relationship between these was hardly fortuitous as both reasonable expressions of the interconnectedness of empirical skill and spiritual belief. Since the most obvious realities were the heavenly bodies with their periodicities and diurnal cycles and the power and fear of sickness it was easy to imagine cosmic forces influencing health and disease, relating eclipses, comets, changes in the lunar phases, etc., to earthly events and health, infirmity and death; but there is another connection between medicine and astronomy which is perhaps more basic. The possibility of accurately predicting events by reading astronomical ciphers, on the one hand, and the possibility of predicting the outcome of a disease for a sick man, on the other, elevated one with such skills to a special status. Hence, the practical efforts of the astrologer-astronomer and the priest-physician not only shaped the responses of the individual and the community, but fulfilled a spiritual need that occupied the life of the community in all of its activities.

We see, then, that by virtue of these techniques and skills the shaman was both unique and exemplary, but only because there could not have been another way. Primitive man's needs were spiritual as well as practical. And he sought to satisfy both in order to maintain his own psychic harmony and his harmony with nature.

The greatest difference between the primitive and the modern man is precisely this; in an age of positive knowledge the sense of spirit has dimmed while the need remains. Man, after all, is always trying to bring his experience into harmony with his cosmic sense. The primitive, without science, was reverent of nature and cosmos; modern man, with science, seeks their domination.

The Way

There is a story told about a yogi who approached the master to inquire as to how he will know when he has met Brahman. The master paused and spoke, "when you have walked across the great river and touched the clouds." The initiate hesitated, then added that he had already done so. The master replied, "then you have answered the question."

The Eastern master has always suggested that existence is absurd and the world of experience is fleeting and illusory. Even time is unreal, a ceaseless becoming, a Thoreau-like "stream to go-a-fishin' in." The world offers neither personal fulfillment nor realization; rather each man is caught in the vortex of Karma, his unchanging destiny. The individual's best hope is renunciation of the world and the passage of the soul through its various transformations until it reaches the timeless "One." Detachment is necessary to remove the pain of living in and involvement with the world. One withdraws to survive. What is more in contrast to our own view, the reality of the sensible world and a moral imperative to make it better? This difference in "world view," the way the Eastern mind and the Western mind comprehend being and existence has been fundamental to the advancement of science. In the West, during the long course of its intellectual growth, the idea of science grew in concert with the evolution of our world view and its particular expression after Christianity.

The growth of Western science can only be appreciated with regard to its conspicuous absence in the East, which directly relates to Eastern philosophy. This is not to say that the Eastern thinker did not believe in any reality, only that his reality was beyond anything touching him in his earthly existence. Western philosophy and Christian thought have some measure of this sense of dualism but Christianity has always taught that both the material world and the spiritual world are real. Indeed, the Christian only achieves the latter through the former. The Eastern mind, on the other hand, viewed the world as something that must be renounced both as reality and as value.

The origins of Hindu philosophy lie in an obscurity related both to the East's geographical and philosophical remoteness from the West. What evidence remains of those origins, however, suggests that a great movement from the highlands of central Asia and the Himalayas, and from the plateaus of the North, occurred in the third or fourth milienium before Christ, populating the great regions of later Indian civilization. These migrations sent fair-skinned peoples west into what is now modern Iran and south into India. By this time two great societies had already formed on the banks of the Indus at MohenjoDaro and Harapa, poppulated by dark-skinned natives. The Aryans conquered these cities and eventually grafted their Aryan culture on to the native one while introducing their own oral tradition, the Vedas.

The Vedas ultimately were to form the basis of India's greatest indigenous philosophy and method of living, Hinduism. The flowering of Hindu civilization, however, did not take place on the banks of the Indus but further East, on the banks of the Brahmaputra and the Ganges. Here the "Vedas" ("hymn" in Sanskrit) were sung and their message spoke to the mysteries of the universe and of the "One" called *Brahman,* the great spiritual essence of the universe. The Vedic poems portrayed man alone in a universe whose truth was discoverable through meditation. Vedic truth results from introspection and intuition rather than from the contemplation of the physical world and Hinduism enunciates a philosophy of monistic idealism, the spiritual unity of the world and the "One," reflecting the Indian bias to synthesis. This had been an approach which, until recently, was subjective and intuitive while the Western attitude has grown increasingly analytic and objective. Obviously, the Eastern view of the physical world and the belief in the chaotic nature of existence was unlikely to inspire an Eastern thinker to make science. Likewise, this devaluation of the world summoned the Indian mystic to pass through his stages of karma, that universal and unforgiving principle of retribution where, as Heschel says, "there is no grace and there is no forgiveness," to reach the "One," Brahman. Yet Karma is a harsh and immutable law which casts a gloomy pessimism over life in the East. There is no escape from karma, only a long sequence of lives until the incubus of, "this mortal coil," is finally cast off. For the Hindu there is no social gospel, nor any value in an effort to develop science or gain positive knowledge as this would only be a ridiculous description of illusory being.

The *Upanishads,* the concluding parts of the Vedas, are the revelation (sutra) spoken by the sages of the Vedic faith. They are mystical illuminations which illustrate the negating spirit of their philosophy. In the Catha Upanishad, for instance, the way to Brahman opens when finally:

> Cease the five sense knowledges, together with the mind, and the intellect stirs not. That they say is the highest course, this they consider as yoga, the firm holding back of the senses. Then one becomes undistracted. Not by speech . . . not by mind, not by sight can he be apprehended (The One). How can he be comprehended otherwise than by one saying he is.[1]

This, "he is," and its magical symbol "Om" present a striking similarity to the Hebrew tetragrammaton YHVH, "I am who am." but Yahweh, unlike all the Vedic deities, is the God who reveals Himself.

Consider the mystical passage in the Mundaka Upanishad, concerning the "Om":

> Taking as a bow the great weapon of the Upanishad, one should put upon it an arrow sharpened by meditation stretching it with a thought directed to the essence . . . The mystic syllable is the bow, the arrow is the self, Atman. Brahman is said to be the mark, by the undistracted man is it to be penetrated.[2]

The undistracted man is the detached man who finds "div," the light (the Sanskrit root for "divinity"). The illumination he seeks is the cosmic consciousness of Atman joined with Brahman. Surely this undistracted man is not a man of science; he is not really a man of this world. Even his self-reflecting consciousness is a distraction.

In the epic period, dating from the sixth century before Christ, the literature of the Hindu developed. The Vedas and the Upanishads, initially a rich and familiar oral tradition, are now written. "The One" gradually takes on a more personal character. The great work of this period is the religious epic, the Mahabharata, in a section of which, the *Bhagavad-Gita,* the world is depicted as the scene of two great antagonisms good and evil. The persistent philosophical dualism is maintained, but something is added. There is a hint that there is a god who is interested in the outcome!

In addition to the epic tradition several heterodox systems developed and sharpened Hindu philosophy. The most reactionary of them was the *Carvaka,* the only Indian system to place any value on the sensible world and the reality of sense perception. Indeed, the Carvaka understood sense perception as the only source of knowledge. The Carvaka taught a sensible world consisting of four elements similar to that in the Empedoclean Greek model. It emphasized the orderly arrangement of the cosmos but taught that since one cannot know the universality of a principle proposition, except through perception, it is impossible to establish any inference, hence it is impossible to gain new knowledge through logic alone. Aristotle, in contrast, accepted *a priori* the "giveness" of universals as independent of perception but known through it, leading to knowledge and an understanding of causality. The Carvaka rejected causality by rejecting the inference, an obviously unpropitious tenet for the development of science.

The greatest of the heterodox systems is Buddhism, a philosophy of supreme renunciation which measures life as a continuous flow of strife through the stages of reincarnation until ultimate release from that universal law of "morality," karma. In its early and less refined form, Hinayana Buddhism, things are illusionary and fleeting; in the more mature Mahayana Buddhism, life becomes a process of attainment. Life is now a stream of becoming and attainment is won by the ascetic who desires nothing. "He would look upon the world as a bubble, look upon it as a mirage. Him who so looks upon this world, the king of death does not see ... Who is the Brahman? You might call a brahman, he who in this world, giving up all craving, wanders about without a home and whom all craving for existence is extinguished."[3]

During the Buddhist formative period, new orthodox systems began to develop in India in opposition to the skepticism of Buddhism. These systems accepted the philosophical and mystical authority of the Vedas while adding their own unique contribution of logical analysis to the Vedic works. They accepted the inference (the Carvaka had denied it) as a valid means of gaining knowledge. The universality of certain first principles was accepted and as making inferential statements and deductive reasoning possible. Yet there was still no attempt at a comprehensive natural philosophy and their logic could only be applied to the meditative exercise.

We can easily see that with these various systems it was hard to imagine a scientific view of reality developing, especially as the very existence of "reality" itself was at issue. The problematical nature of material things and the objects of sense experience forced Indian thought away from a rational study of concrete reality, even though there were some advances in astronomy and mathematics. Indian astronomy described solar and lunar events and developed a calendar and some mathematical explanations for the periodicity of extraterrestrial phenomena. The Indians were also the first to develop the decimal system and elementary geometry. Despite these advances they never started on the road to science and the serious investigation of the physical world because Indian cosmology and philosophy remained entirely transcendent.

Chinese philosophical developments were similar to those in India in that reality was looked upon as being intensely psychological, with the difference that the Chinese had a more dualistic view of existence. Like the Indian the Chinese approached the understanding of reality and the illumination of existence through the solitary way of meditation. In Taoism, for instance, the seeker of the "way" arrives at insights and answers to the cosmic mysteries and his own life experiences through a soul search that is intensely spiritual. At the same time it is practical, allowing one to "deal" with life situations by practiced inaction. This is not the absolute indifference of the Hindu, but a principle, acting only when an action will have a salutory or beneficial effect for the one acting. Either the act will have a meaningful effect or the act, in the first place, is superfluous, in which case inaction is preferred.

Taoism is one of the two great indigenous Chinese systems, the other being Confucianism. Taoism owes a great deal to Lao Tzu, one of the first great teachers of the Taoist mysteries and the way of the Tao. Lao Tzu wrote the *Tao Te Ching* in which, in addition to the way, there was a doctrine of the "te," virtue, and a doctrine of the "pu," the teaching of the self. Taoism's formation in the fifth century before Christ paralleled developments in Buddhism and Confucianism, but Taoism was less introspective than Buddhism and in some respects similar to Confucianism in that it preached the utility of the suppression of desire. Both were personal philosophies of contemplation as well as methods from which rules and norms of social conduct could be defined.

The *I Ching* formed a base for all of the indigenous Chinese systems; Taoism, Confucianism, Chinese Buddhism and Chinese Zen. In the *I Ching*, which dates back at least one to two millenia before Christ, the principles of the five elements, earth, wood, fire, water and metal, and the principle of the integrated forces of the yin and the yang are developed. The yin and the yang are not opposing principles whereby one is to be overcome at the sacrifice of the other, rather they are complementary forces to be found in a harmonious interaction. One can not fail to see the parallels between the doctrine of the five elements and the yin and yang and something that we will meet in the development of Greek thought where the four elements are matched with the Empedoclean doctrine of love and strife. Like the Empedoclean doctrine, the yin and the yang is dualistic, but this dualism is meant to be affirmed as a synthesis in the completion of the individual and his existence.

Perhaps the most inscrutable of the Eastern philosophies is Zen. Zen, which flowered in Japan and in other parts of the Far East, was originally the product of the interaction of Buddhism with Taoism providing the basis for an intensely personal encounter with oneself. Zen is neither a philosophy nor a system of conduct whose rules can be applied to society. It simply states that what is, is for each individual at each moment. The conduct of one's life is a high art and each human being experiences life uniquely. The exhilaration of living cannot be shared with another, certainly not as a general method of affirmation or denial. Zen is an extreme merging of conscious and subconscious, without the self-consciousness Western psychoanalysis would demand. It is, at the same time, the experience of oneness and totality. There is no call for the flight of the soul out of the body to a transcendent order, but a call for everything to converge in the soul, unfettered by any sense of the soul being separated from existence or hindered by other psyches.

Zen is replete with self-contradictory koans (statements). It argues against the principles of reason and for an individual discovery, one's own way through. This is not unlike the approach one must take to the *I Ching, The Book of Changes,* which is also intensely personal. Each hexagram in the *I Ching* is meant to illustrate a problem and the possibilities for solution. Both the problem and the solution come from the depths of the soul. The *I Ching* speaks but one can only act on what one hears, and what one hears, of course, has an internal dynamic which makes the solution different for each one who approaches the book. It is by this personal, reflective method that the wisdom of the *I Ching* is revealed. For the Hindu, the Buddhist, the Taoist or the followers of Confucius, all converges on the self and, as the self finds itself, it defines its own reality. Rationalism and objective knowledge is not possible, as it would be absurd to develop a general theory about illusory being. Western thought, on the other hand, is causally oriented, looking both for objective meanings and their refinement into bodies of knowledge that can be principles for right conduct or scientific understanding but can in either case be lifted from the particular to the general. Thus we see the ultimate failure of the scientific impulse in the East and India. Neither India nor China developed a science based on causality and rational explanations or theories of phenomena. This is the very point of an examination of their philosophies. To display the Judeo-Christian world view and its notion of a rationally created universe, knowable, understandable and good because created, over and against a world neither good nor knowable, is to provide a fundamental explanation for the Western achievement.

The Way to Health

Eastern medicine, including the Egyptian and Babylonian Near Eastern medicine, was informed by Eastern philosophical, religious and cultural attitudes. Medicine mixed a good deal of the spiritual and the magical with the empirical which also presented theories of disease or illness based on the philosophical views of man and reality. Disease was often viewed in a moral context, one's ethical behavior and respect for custom and tradition, for instance, had great bearing on health in the Chinese and Indian systems. More general philosophical or spiritual thinking also influenced ideas about causality in disease, those factors that were thought to be involved with illness or death. Many of these, such as the interplay of Yin and Yang or the balance of humours were more spiritual notions than physiological ones in contrast to Greek thinking especially after Hippocrates, Aristotle and Galen when the theories were primarily physiological. Nonetheless, Eastern medicine was often empirically sound, passing the test of reproducible successes, so in some respects it advanced as a practical art further than the spiritual definitions of illness and healing related to Eastern philosophy might have suggested.

Indian and Chinese physicians practiced with exquisite regard for ritual and the uncertain and coincidental nature of all events. Much of the ritual, of course, was bound to religious customs and was not primarily meant to be therapeutic in a physical sense, rather as religious practices they also incidentally provided bodily relief. The traditional Oriental emphasis on diet, ritual bathing, massage, breathing exercises, physical discipline, climatology and meteorology is not unlike the similar emphasis which we will see in Hippocratic medicine, the difference being that neither Hindu nor Chinese healers developed a theory of disease based on strict physical causality or used specific therapies separate in a scientific way.

An example of this is the Chinese and Hindu practice of pulse examination. This art included an examination of the pulse in the forearm and of all the great vessels, an exercise taking many hours, providing hundreds of descriptions of pulse characteristics in various disease states. It is unclear, however, if the Chinese actually appreciated the circulation of the blood and the heart as the blood pump. The Chinese drew the association between the pulse and the vital principle, noting changes in the pulse in various diseases and its absence immediately prior to death. Obviously the cessation of the pulse and breathing at death suggested that they are the very essence of life, the *vita anima*, so even without a theory of the circulation the character of the pulse still had great prognostic value and spiritual implications. We can also imagine the benefits to the patient such pulse touching carried with it. Even today the first act of the physician at the bedside is the examination of the pulse and it remains an exercise that has great psychological value, suggesting an intimacy with illness that harkens back to that very ancient practice.

Indian medicine, like the Chinese, was inseparable from philosophy. The brahman was a healer, a religious figure and an astronomer. He performed elaborate bedside rituals, verbal therapies, massages, baths, often accompanied by recitation of the vedas or the wisdom of the sages. You must remember that for the Indian disease was punishment; it had moral and retributive value. This was also true in China, Egypt and in the Babylonian construction, so that the priest occupied a central role in healing. As empirical knowledge and healing skills developed, the priest was less in evidence and a high degree of specialization ensued and in later periods in both China and Egypt we find that each organ, each disease, each remedy, has its own specialist. Finally, physicians became civil servants, functionaries in the highly bureaucratic systems peculiar to the East.

India did not produce any single noteworthy medical text or compendium, but China had a great work, *The Yellow Emperor's Classic of Internal Medicine* or the *Huang Ti Nei Ching*. This work, initially compiled as early as the fourth or fifth century before Christ, was a "tao of healing," emphasizing the spiritual aspects of health and disease—the five elements and the ying and the yang, and the interaction and balance of these in the interior milieu. The yin and the yang, in the medical context, were analogous to the balanced but opposing physiological components of the autonomic nervous system elucidated much later in Western medicine. Consistent with the yin and yang the Chinese had separated organs into systems, the solid or yang organs; lungs, spleen, heart, kidneys and liver; four hollow or yin organs; bladder, and the alimentary tract or organs of digestion and the gall bladder. This arrangement was not strictly "causal" in the physiological sense that we understand in Western medicine, it was more a basis for a philosophical explanation of health and disease.

Each organ system, in addition to its principle "yin" or "yang," had a topographical representation which formed the basis for the ancient Chinese practice of acupuncture. This art developed around a complex system of skin mapping, correlating external reference markers to their respective organ systems. The topographical elements, the principle meridians, were considered functional representations of the interior and part of the harmonious interaction of yin and yang. Stimulation along the appropriate meridian lines led to the activation of the various organs, the particular type of organ stimulated, be it solid or hollow, then determining in which direction restoration would proceed.

The important parallels between acupuncture topography and organ representation in the Western concept of the nervous systems suggests the empirical basis of acupuncture techniques in Chinese medicine. In addition, modern medicine has developed an explanation for acupuncture success based on two facts: the presence of electrical potentials over the entire skin surface; the relation between the nervous innervation of surface zones and internal organs; the dermatome patterns responsible for referred pain elucidated by Head and McKenzie in the nineteenth century.

Acupuncture must also be understood as having great psychological merit. Its efficacy is in good measure related to the expectations of the patient who is aware of its long tradition in culture; it is thus often self-validating. There is one interesting statement in the *Nei Ching* about this. The Emperor asks Chi Po (his prime minister) what is necessary to achieve good results. Chi Po answers, "This is the way of acupuncture; if a man's vitality and energy do not propel his own will, his disease cannot be cured." How often and emphatically will that wisdom be reaffirmed by the wisest physicians with regard to all methods of healing.

Both Indian and Chinese medicine grew to be administered disciplines. Supervision of medicine and surgery required codes of behavior for surgeons, herbalists and all of the other specialists. There were specified measures for a breech of ethics or poor results. The Indian *Codes of Manu* emphatic on punishments for malpractice and the Chinese *Chou Li* first ennumerated the classes of physicians and specialists, their duties under the supervision of the chief physician and the disciplinary procedures for malfeasance. Many surgeons forfeited a finger, hand or arm for degrees of negligence, or for bad results when a fee was taken (Thank God that's over!). The *Chou Li* manual was consistent with the Chinese interest in administration and public works. After all, the Chinese have given us the very model of the civil servant, the Mandarin, the perfect bureaucrat who maintained his position first through success on competitive examination, thereafter through corruption, a fine art among pious Buddhist bureaucrats.

Indian and Chinese medicine made advances in surgery as well as healing methods. The Hindus practiced cosmetic nose surgery. They were also accomplished lithotomists and tumor surgeons. They knew the principle behind ligatures and sutures. Similar surgery for wounds, fractures and cosmesis was performed in China and both cultures made great strides in hygiene as an outgrowth of their efforts in public works, agriculture and water control. At one point Indian medicine had a theory of disease based on the humours and concepts of fever with its evolution through stages or crises very similar to that which we would see with the Hippocratic physicians later. Even the *Nei Ching* anticipated Hippocratic thought on the environment, air, water, places and diet and regimen, suggesting some attempts at theories of causality in disease, although most medical thinking in the East was still philosophical rather than scientific.

Egyptian medicine was related to Eastern medicine in its organization and its concepts about disease in relation to Egyptian religion. Egyptian medicine was primarily the business of the state as Egypt had developed the most heirarchical and complex administrative apparatus in the Near East. Egypt also evolved into a theocratic state in which the Pharoah, at first only a representative of the gods, was finally himself a god. As the Pharoah grew in his "godliness" the bureaucracies swelled to serve him in architecture, public works, temple and pyramid building and the practice of medicine. This medicine was highly charged with magic and superstition. Initially, it was overseen by the priests of the temples, later it became more specialized so that physicians replaced the priests. Their medicine contained the usual herbal and surgical approaches but the Egyptians progressed further in particular areas such as embalming with resins, spices, and oils to forestall decomposition. The Egyptian skill in developing antibacterials carried over to their use in cosmetics as well. The eye paints, body lotions, perfumes and salves possessed some antibacterial and antifungal properties, evidence of the chemical skills the Egyptians possessed. There is also one curious note about Egyptian medicine and hygiene. The Egyptians were the most compulsive enema users in the ancient world, a practice consistent with their view that the anus was the center of death and decay. Even the action of the sacred bird of the pharoahs, the long beaked ibis washing its anus with its beak, provided a reminder which hardly went unnoticed.

The ancient orders of Egyptian priest-physicians anticipated the growth of the Asclepian priestly healing cults in Greece before the emergence of the Hippocratics. The Egyptian priests superintended state medicine and closely regulated the conduct of physicians and the medical schools in the Empire. Originally, the priests were the initiates into sacred mysteries of the Egyptian religion and the interpreters of astrological signs. These offices conferred special status and power in the conduct of healing and hygienic practices. In time the priests claimed those privileges for their heirs as followers of Imhotep, the Egyptian Asclepius, the god of healing and medicine. The theocratic character of Egyptian society assured the priests preeminence but as medicine became more specialized more physicians entered the art.

Specialization brought experts in the use of herbals and minerals, cosmetic and traumatic surgery, public health and preparation of the body for the elaborate Egyptian funerary rites, though some of this was performed by non-physicians. Egyptian specialization advanced to the point that physicians often limited themselves to one disease, surgery on one organ or supervision of one facet of the elaborate state programs in hygiene and public works. Inevitably, the expansion of the bureaucracy followed and physicians came under the close supervision of chief physicians. Codes were established which provided for punishment of malpractice and performance review. Procedural guides defined the role of physicians, their assistants and technicians in public works. The Egyptians, much like the Romans, were compulsive builders and many facilities were erected for health and physical culture and water control and waste disposal facilities; huge public baths and hospital-like buildings were constructed under the supervision of the state bureaucracy which regulated the medical personnel involved.

Religion was a constraining influence in all aspects of Egyptian life and the motive force for their achievements. Nonetheless, as with every culture social decay arrived and the religious forms grew increasingly illegitimate, the government more despotic, and medicine more crude. Egyptian medicine became "a trade of sorcerers, drug vendors and charlatans," so that their greatly respected practice of medicine throughout the ancient world finally withered as preeminence passed to the Greeks.

Babylonian-Chaldean medicine was similar to Egyptian medicine and a good deal of it was in the hands of the priest caste. The Babylonians and Chaldeans were enthusiastic astrologers and virtually all of their treatments were conducted with astrological considerations. They believed that celestial events bore directly on health and that the constellations directly influenced one's life from birth to death. They made use of divination from the study of internal organs, particularly the liver, which was considered the source of the blood and anima. Dream interpretation was a developed art. Dreams, like celestial events, guided the conduct of individual and social life. Specialization did not approach that in Egyptian medicine nor did the priests ever loosen their hold on medicine. Religion, medicine and magic never separated, limiting the growth of empirical medicine.

There were no general theories of disease perhaps explaining the heavy emphasis on magic and astrology. Like Indian, Chinese and Egyptian medicine, however, Babylonian-Chaldean medicine developed into a state function with codes of conduct and statutes bearing on incompetents, including the Code of Hammurabi, a Babylonian king who codified the law two millenia before Christ. Likewise, the Babylonian priest-caste dominated medicine and law and promoted specialization and rigid guidelines for performance of specific healing functions, many of which were later delegated to physicians who were not priests.

All of the Eastern cultures shared some common features in regard to medicine; priests played a dominant role, medical organization became bureaucratic, and medical theory remained primarily spiritual. Humoral theories and causal thinking, when they appear, are still related to spiritual forces in nature and its changes, empirical success in the herbal, mineral and surgical therapies notwithstanding. Eastern medicine was not scientific in the sense that the Greeks began to develop it, primarily because the Eastern philosophies did not undertake the examination of natural phenomena in themselves, separate from the spiritual element. That step was taken by the Greeks.

The Greeks and Science

Medicine was the most important and perhaps most developed science in Greece. Greek physicians were the first to study disease from the aspect of material causality separate from spiritual categories and examined through etiology, sign, symptom and prognosis. In doing this the Greeks emphasized those now familiar elements of the scientific approach; observation, analysis, synthesis and deduction. Such methods in the healing arts are traditionally associated with the Hippocratics but many other Greeks presented general theories of disease.

Greek medicine was an outgrowth of the Greek passion for philosophical inquiry and a desire to develop a natural philosophy. Because of the special interest in medicine, many Greek philosophers were physicians and held opinions regarding disease consistent with their understanding of a rational order in nature. Both as philosophers and as scientific theorists they sought the unifying principle(s) behind the order and regularity of natural and celestial events. These efforts were already in evidence with the pre-Socratics and intensified with Plato and Aristotle, though Plato's science was limited to the political realm. Aristotle, on the other hand, pursued many sciences, including biology, becoming the foremost biologist in the Greek world.

Greek science and medicine began with the pre-Socratics in Ionia, Asia Minor and in Southern Italy and Sicily and the historical figure usually cited as the first philosopher (obviously he wasn't) is Thales. He is "the representative man" in this new intellectual voyage. Thales was the first thinker to seek an explanation for phenomena not in myth or fate but in phenomena themselves. Thales taught that the unifying principle of "kosmos" is water and that water is the primary constituent element in all matter. Physical changes come about as the result of the changes in phases of this primary element, water and ice. This intellectual leap of Thales, which left animism behind and founded natural philosophy, was as great a leap as the leap from classical physics to quantum physics in our time, a qualitative difference in thought from all that had preceded. After Thales, other Greek philosophers followed with their own theories.

Anaximander of Miletus claimed that the cosmos was an organized whole with a concrete arrangement of things in time. Anaximander's thinking influenced early Greek medicine and physics considerably. His cosmos was a balance of opposites, cold and heat, dry and wet, dark and light, a balance serving as the basis for his theory of disease, a view ultimately enlarged upon by Alcmaeon and the Hippocratics. *Heraclitus* thought the first element in the cosmos is a fire and that remains constant through all change in nature and cosmos. One element or physical body may change into another through fire by the purest transmutations possible but fire itself is immutable.

Heraclitus' theory of change disturbed a school of philosophers in southern Italy. This group, the *Eleatics,* was quickly taking speculative thought to new heights. Indeed, they may be cited as the first victims of the excesses of reason. The major Eleatics, Parmenidies and Zeno, argued that if anything were changing, certainly if all things were constantly changing, then nothing could remain of their original. Thus nothing, in fact, could "be" unless it remained as it "is." "Being" cannot be changing; "being" must be immutable, permanent and therefore motion cannot "be" since this would imply change. Consider the arrow in flight, said Zeno; at an instant in time it must be at a specific locus in space, i.e., it must be at rest. So, Zeno argued, why make a theory of motion where there is only a body in an infinite series at rest? Now this intellectual conceit was a great deceit, it denied the testimony of the senses. Obviously this was reasoning carried to an absurd extreme, yet the history of thought is not without its absurdities. The danger is, as Pascal would later say, that excessive rationalism always ends in the assassination of reason itself.

The absurdity of the Eleatic position required a rational response. Leucippus and Democritus answered the dilemma posed by the Parmenidean doctrine of permanence and Zeno's paradoxes by stating that behind the diversity of physical realities there is an underyling unity of indivisible and invisible atoms, miniatures of the material beings they compose. These atoms combine in groups of different sizes and shapes to constitute the elements. This doctrine was a modification of the views of another thinker, *Anaxagoras,* who also believed in "elementary" particles which, however, were not indivisible. Anaxagoras had also introduced the concept of "nous" (mind) as an ordering principle of the cosmos. Mind is the regulator of the movement of the particles of matter. *Leucippus,* however, held that motion is an inherent property of these atoms. *Democritus,* the pupil of Leucippus, emphasized the unity of all things through the atoms. He noted that we can have knowledge of concrete beings themselves because these extrude countless atoms which are their miniatures. These impinge on the senses and cause the "soul" atom to resonate inside the observer, granting him perception.

The Pre-Socratics were not only engaged in these speculations, they involved themselves in medical theory-making and the development of healing methods based on them as well. Thus many of the prominent Pre-Socratics were physician-philosophers and among their most representative figures was Empedocles of Agrigentium.

Empedocles lived in the first half of the fifth century B.C., about the time that Zeno and Parmenides were being "unreasonable". He was a practicing physician who prescribed for patients through diet and regimen and made diagnoses based on his configuration of illness as a dysharmony of the internal milieu, the disturbances of the four elements: earth, fire, air, and water. He understood disease as a process involving the mixture of these elements within and their arrangement outside the sick man. He also outlined a theory of the evolution of the universe from primeval material through the alternating triumph of love and strife, antithetical forces which shape material being and spiritual reality. This notion that the universe evolves from primeval material was a theory held by many Ionian and Egyptian thinkers. Empedocles also developed a theory of the circulation of the blood and respiration and even demonstrated that atmospheric air was distinct from the "void."

Empedocles' four elements may actually have been borrowed from the Egyptians and were similar to the three primeval elements of Hindu cosmology. Their application to medicine was direct, however, in the theory of "isonomia," the harmonious balance between the four elements and the soul principle within the person. This doctrine was developed more freely by *Alcmaeon* of Croton and Democedes, a Pythagorean physician in the service of the court of Darius. Alcmaeon, more systematic than Democedes, taught that health was a good mixture, *isonomia,* of the hot and cold, wet and dry, dark and light and the other elements. When these were in proper proportion and in harmony with the psyche (the soul), the individual enjoyed "sophrosyne," the temperate accord of all the elements of his being. Alcmaeon was also a working physician; he prescribed diet and ritual bathing. He took notice of climatological and meterological factors in disease and the incidences of different diseases during different seasons. He was among the first to perform extensive animal dissections and was the first to trace the optic nerves to the chiasma by removing the eyeballs. He sought to find the seat of the soul in the brain and viewed it as the center of mental disturbances. Before Alcmaeon the heart had been considered the seat of emotion and sensation. Alcmaeon also elaborated a theory of the phylogeny of plants and did work on plant germination that antedated modern botanical research by two millenia.

Little is known about the personality of Pythagoras, the founder of the brotherhood that Alcmaeon studied with. Pythagoras had left the island of Samos because of an unfavorable political situation and established a school in Crotona in Southern Italy. There in his mystical medical group he taught number cosmology. This cosmology defined reality through the geometrical quality of material objects, a geometric principle based in number. The Pythagorean notion of number was also closely related to music. They had recognized the strict numerical relationship between pitch and the geometrically precise units of length on the musical string. This piece of "scientific intuition" helped Pythagoras solidify his notion that number was the basis for all phenomena. At the same time the association between number and music was an explanation of the magic of music coextensive with the magic of number. Thus, the Pythagoreans could apply the magic of music and the science of number together in their healing work. Different tones and sounds of music were presented to the patient with the same blending that a concoction of herbs would be given. The musical blends were intended to soothe the sick man by charming his psyche and moving his soul.

Music therapy and word charms had been practiced by healers throughout the ancient world. All had recognized the magical, curative power of words and used them to expel the "daimons," the malevolent spirits of illness. Empedocles had recognized the curative power of words and the writings of Alcmaeon and Plato (*The Charmides*) add further testimony to the widespread use of magical logotherapy in the classical world. The Pythagoreans also employed the usual dietary therapies, fasting, ritualistic bathing and meditation, all evidence of Eastern influences. Pythagoras had travelled to Egypt and perhaps further East and was initiated into the mystical rites of the Egyptian fertility and generative cults. He learned many of their methods and practices and combined these with the methods of the Orphic and Delphic cults, including the notion of a psyche that dwelled outside the body because it separated from the soul at death. Pythagoras divided this soul into three parts, the thymous, nous and phrenes, and said that health was the proper harmony of the three. The internal harmony could be enhanced by music, diet, dream satisfaction and meditation, promoting the health and stability of the psyche and soma together.

Pythagorean thought, in sum, held the cosmos to be mathematically ordered and in sympathy with the psyche, while holding many ideas related to Orphic dualism and the idea of two worlds which matured in Plato's philosophy. Pythagorean dualism continued in the Platonic cosmology, especially as it is discussed in the *Timaeus,* and in early Christian metaphysics derived from the Neo-platonic world view. The Pythagorean unity, on the other hand, unity through number/mathematics, served as one basis for subsequent development in the natural sciences, especially the astronomy and physics of Kepler, Galileo and Newton. One other curious thing about number, mathematics and music comes to mind. The relation between music and mathematics seems never to have been expressed in the same way in the Eastern tradition. The identity between music and number was not made and number/mathematics was never the basis of an understanding of the cosmos. Perhaps this mathematical awareness was an important part of the West's heritage in science based on an ordered cosmos, and its absence a reason for the failure of science in the East.

The work of the early Greek philosophers underscores their interest in the study of being as being, an attempt to both unify and analyze natural phenomena. This undertaking could not have proceeded without a movement toward separating being and the qualities of being from their previous spirituality. But the spiritual essence of a controlling principle in the cosmos remained indispensible to their cosmology as the "ultimate" first reality. The concept of nous, the directing intelligence, grew in importance as the creative force differentiating the material world from its ordering activity. This nous was not a personal creator like the Christian God, yet we are not entitled to say that nous did not in any sense anticipate that moral executor, and the Platonic cosmology which followed with its Demiurgos comes closer to the idea of a creating God. One thing is certain, however. Pre-Socratic natural philosophy was an inquiry into nature and its inherent order and rationality. This was the Greek "physis," the coherent world of being, the study of which in its material reality would become *physics* while its management in the art and science of the sick man became the basis for the theory and practice of medicine as *physic.*

The physis was understood in the context of a metaphysical world view occupied with the subject of being as being. The similarities between Pythagorean (and Platonic thought), on the one hand, and Near Eastern and Indian cosmology and philosophy, on the other, suggests a substantial amount of borrowing from the East. Yet Greek physics broke from the mystery philosophies, both the homegrown, such as the Eleusian and Delphic and those which they were familiar with through contacts with Egypt and Chaldea. The break was evident when the Greeks undertook the study of material reality as a proper subject in itself. This decisive intellectual activity, begun in the sixth century in Iona, was important in the history of science because this method was necessary to know the physis. The important point for our story is precisely this; the early Greek "physicists" believed that the world and cosmos were knowable, i.e., comprehensible. Order prevailed in the multiplicity of things and unity in the diversity in change. The next step, with Plato and Aristotle, was the more specific reference to an ordering principle and more complete theories of knowledge.

Plato, one of the most important figures in Western thought, taught in his Academy in Athens in the first half of the fourth century B. C. He joined elements of Eastern philosophy with Pythagorean number cosmology and added his own theories of the nature of reality and the transcendent order of genuine knowledge. Plato was primarily a metaphysician. His interest, that is, was in the informing idea behind the material universe. He characterized the world of the senses as a plurality of imperfect beings, substances, replicas of their pure forms in a Noumenal world. This transcendent world of true being included both the exemplars of all material things as well as the subjects of intellection and abstraction such as goodness, virtue, justice and love. These universals, the ideas or forms, are the province of the soul, mind or "Nous." They are timeless, perfected and archetypical. On the other hand, Plato's sensible world was not just an illusion, maya, as it was for the brahman but a world that could be studied to lead the intellect to the universals.

Buddhism, you will recall, is the model philosophy of negation, a denial of the sensible world both ontologically and in the Buddhist's ethical witness. For the Buddhist the self and the road to the one and indivisible transcend the immediate in time to meet the ultimate in timelessness. Plato made life a quest for transcendent truth as well, since a knowledge of universals was true knowledge, i.e. scientific knowledge. But Plato also knew that the universals are present in individual things though individual things could not be a source of true knowledge in themselves. True knowledge was a share in the idea of the creative nous, the intellectual force in the cosmos, through the activity of the soul. Likewise, Plato's immortality is a state wherein one possesses the world of the good after death because the soul, pure form, survives matter, its substance. These notions were shared by the Pythagoreans and other Greek cosmologists and were borrowed by the neo-Platonists, the early Christian fathers and some medievalists.

Plato believed that it was necessary to cast off the armature of the senses to know the ideas. In *The Phaedo* he states that "he attains to the purest knowledge who goes to each with the mind alone, he who has got rid of eyes, ears and so to speak of the whole body. . . . This is finally realized, of course, after death, for then the soul will exist in herself alone."[1] Yet we should recognize a contradiction "in men studying to live as nearly as they can in a state of death yet repining when it comes upon them." Thus the life of the senses and world of objects has meaning and by the apprehension of their particulars a man will have some understanding of the universals. There is a theological implication to Plato's teaching as it at once incorporates immortality and the world of pure being into the ultimate object of life. In the *Phaedo* Plato attributes an innate knowledge of essences to the soul, and recollection of these ideas from a soul life prior to corporality, a doctrine of reminiscences akin to that of the Hindus and Pythagoreans.

Plato's metaphysical views crystallize in the *Timaeus* where "Demiurge" is introduced as the symbol of nous, the universal mind, governing principle of the universe. The "Demiurge" is a conscious force, the ideal good creating the material world of particular things from their models in the world of pure forms. Plato, however, distinguishes this creator from the universals which have an objective existence in the ideal world as well as particular, thus qualified, existences in material things. Plato does not discuss how much of the essence of things is arrived at by soul reminiscence and how much by perception, thought and intuition but he does present the material world as proper subject for rational investigation, even if this cannot provide complete knowledge, i.e. knowledge of the ideals.

Plato taught that the forms (the ideas) exist in geometric arrangements so that number becomes the unifying principle in Plato's cosmos as it did in the Pythagoreans'. The primacy assigned to number and mathematics by both systems stresses the jointly held belief in the logic of the cosmos, a belief which legitimized astronomy as a scientific pursuit. The periodicity of cosmic events and the rhythm of solar and lunar changes reveal the order of the cosmos. Human reason uses number to discover this order and to rationalize events in the heavens through astronomy. In the *Epinomis* Plato states "that the apparently mazy movements of the heavenly bodies conform to mathematical law and so express the wisdom of God."[2] In that, I suspect, lies an explanation for man's age old fascination with astrology and astronomy.

Plato defined knowledge as the knowledge of ideal forms, those archetypes of being which are known through a primary act of the soul. A science of the physical world, per se, for Plato was not possible, at least not as a science of natural causes sufficient unto itself. Unlike Aristotle who investigated nature to understand the laws that govern change, movement and causality in the physical world, Plato limited "scientific" methods to ordering the political arrangement and ethical conduct of the state, an effort to make a science of political economy.

Plato had an obvious interest in medicine, though I must say this was not born of a scientific urge like that of Aristotle or the Hippocratics. Plato recognized the primary role accorded to medicine among the Greeks of his time and he often alluded to the methods of the physician in his dialogues, even drawing medical analogies to other areas of thought. In the *Phaedo* he notes that medicine must be a subject of the whole man and that healing must be aimed at the soul and in *The Charmides,* Socrates discusses the word charm (epode) with Critias:

> For all good and evil whether in the body or in human nature originates . . . in the soul, so you must begin by curing the soul, that is the first thing, and the cure, my dear friend, has to be effected by the use of certain charms and these charms are fair words. By them temperance (sophrosyne) is implanted in the soul and where temperance is, there health is speedily given, not only to the head, but to the whole body. The great error of our day in the treatment of the human body is that physicians' separate the soul from the body.[3]

In the *Phaedrus,* Plato compares rhetoric to medicine as both are directed to the soul, the one to persuade and the other to heal; and Socrates states that

> rhetoric is like medicine and that is because medicine has to define the nature of the body and rhetoric that of the soul . . . the rhetorician who teaches his pupil to speak scientifically should set forth the nature of that being to which he addresses his speeches and this I conceive to be the soul.[4]

The *Phaedrus* shows Plato's view of medicine as a soul stirring exercise where the good words of the physician are directed to the soul as an act of persuasion, a rhetoric for cure. Thus we see Plato's notion of healing connects back to the methods of the shaman, the medicine man, the temple priest and the pre-Hippocratic Greek physician who recognized the great value of logotherapy.

Through a long and circuitous history this emphasis on the word in healing connects Plato to modern psychotherapy and the "talking cure." Plato had an implicit sense of the noetic status of words. Heidegger, in our own day, reaffirms this: "man takes his stand in language and speaks from there."[5] Language is thought and the "ek-sistence" of man is the extension of individual personality to the outside through language. In our time Heidegger's philosophy of language imparts new meaning to the dialogue between the patient and the physician, recognizing the role of language in the phenomenology of disease and healing, an idea Plato and the ancients well understood.

The philosophers' interest in medicine from the pre-Socratics to Plato, as we have seen, was not primary, or primarily directed toward the practical task of the care of the sick man. Nonetheless, while the Pre-Socratics and the students at Plato's Academy continued their intellectual dialectics one Greek came forward to distinguish himself as a bedside doctor and honor his profes-

sion with his sense of the nobility of its task. It is no wonder that the Hippocratic oath remained for twenty centuries the solemn pledge of the doctor, and
a tragedy for our time that medicine no longer sees its relevance. Let us go
with that doctor and observe the Greek medical mind in theory and in
practice.

The time is somewhere late in the fifth century B.C. and a master observer
of disease is aside the bed of his patient. The doctor is Hippocrates of Cos, the
patient the victim of one of the many infectious diseases, sick with fever and
loss of fluids, weakened by the lack of food. The master approaches calmly to
inquire of his patient about the circumstances of the illness, for he himself
had taught that

> by attending to the general nature of all and the peculiar nature of
> each individual to the disease, the patient and the applications, to
> the person who applies them as that makes a difference for better or
> for worse, to the whole constitution of the season, to the state of
> the heavens, the nature of the country, to the patient's conserva-
> tion, manners, taciturnity, thoughts, sleep and dreams, to all of his
> symptoms, from these and their consequences, we must form our
> judgement.[6]

He consulted the astrological signs, season of the year and meteorological
events. He considered the air, winds and waters and the diseases peculiar to
the region or city where the patient lived. He did not ignore the emotional
state of the patient and he carefully gauged his responses, but neither did
he rest his case solely on the answers. He observed his patient—his color,
the moisture and texture of his skin, his physiognomy and expression, his
breathing, pulse and fever.

The master was intimate with the many faces of disease. Early in his career
he had made careful note of the histories left by the sick in the healing temples
which described symptoms and cures. He carried his bedside observations to
all of his new patients, comparing and analyzing, attempting to group regularly occuring events and patient histories into categories. He had been
thoroughly familiar with the work and writings of other physicians. He was
scholarly and ethical but he also knew his limitations. He had written of his
failures in diagnosis and of his inaccuracies in prognosis, but those admis-
sions only found him more esteemed.

Now, once again at the bedside, after careful questioning and examination,
he is ready to present his findings, the "physic," natural phenomena in disease. He has found an explanation and told his patient and his students, as he
had said "not thereby to impress but to teach." He had weighed the findings

in the framework of the prevalent theories, the disturbances of the humours and the imbalance and dysharmony of the elements. But he was not a dogmatist, for him theory and praxis fit together to the ultimate goal, the relief of the patient before him. He had studied well all of the causes of the distempers, fever, knowing that many of the acute fevers would run a course through stages terminating by crisis. He knew that many other fevers lasted longer but with certain periodicities within their course. He was familiar with diet and could recommend a proper mix of herbs and minerals. He knew when to administer fluids and when to withhold them. He knew the method of bleeding but was judicious in its application.

Hippocrates often observed the patient for the first several days of illness. He would not force fluids or bleed indiscriminately, thus allowing for the body to expel morbid matter on its own. His ministrations were carefully thought out, they were temperate and avoided excess for, as he noted, "no less mischief happens to a man from unreasonable depletion than from repletion."[7] He counseled as to prognosis. He saw symptoms in repetition as a way of making the prediction as to outcome. No doubt this was a source of assurance to the patient and further evidence of the power of the physician, should he be proven correct. He had noted, for instance, that the patient with fever, should he have "sweats about the neck, respiration interrupted in its expulsion of air frequent and large, expressions of eyelids dreadful, these are indications of strong delirium and such patients shall only die."[8]

Hippocrates was an illustrious representative of medicine, considerate of the patient and respectful of the powers of disease. He left his wisdom in his writings and carefully framed in them the principles of the proper practice of medicine. He noted, for instance, that he looked upon it as being a

> great part of the art to be able to judge properly what had been written, for he who knows and makes proper use of these things will not commit any great mistake. Whatever disease will be protracted and end in death and whatever will be protracted and end in recovery, which disease of an acute nature will end in recovery. From these it is easy to know the order of the critical days and prognosticate from them accordingly. To a person who is skilled in these things it is easy to know to whom, when and how elements ought to be administered.[9]

Hippocrates has been acclaimed the father of medicine. In truth, without diminishing his status, he was greatly influenced by the thought of his period and the desire among Greek speculative philosophers to arrive at natural explanations. His medicine showed obvious similarities to that of the schools of southern Italy, Sicily and Cnidos. Pythagorean influence in astronomy, mathematics and medicine had been dispersed throughout the Greek world and among those Pythagoreans, Alcmaeon and Philolaos stood out as physicians who influenced him. Both had approached clinical medicine with regard to natural causes prior to Hippocrates' writings. Empedocles of Agrigentium is mentioned in Hippocrates' work, as is Democritus, the atomist, and other physicians including his father, Heracleides. Hippocrates, in fact, came from a noted medical family said to have had several generations of membership in the Aesculapian circle. From all these he gained knowledge and brought others theories into his notions of disease. He made the scientific element a necessary part of the art of the good physician.

Hippocratic medicine was not without its errors, however, and perhaps the greatest fault of the Coan school, and other schools after Hippocrates, was the gradual debasement of verbal psychotherapy. Pedro Entralgo has pointed out the importance attached to verbal theory prior to Hippocrates. The Pythagorean school made use of verbal healing and the word charm, combining it with music therapy. Plato made special mention of the relationship between medicine and rhetoric, noting that the therapeutic word speech should be subtly recommended to the character and state of mind of the patient, even before the application of a specific remedy. Plato also noted the importance of the patient's trust in and receptivity to the healing word and the insights regarding our notion of "placebo" are striking. Unhappily, the Hippocratics accorded the verbal mode a diminished status in the therapeutic setting and it passed into a secondary role in bedside medicine. After all, the physician who acquired rational and causally oriented therapy was not in need of shamanistic modes. Thus, the excessive logotherapy of the primitive was replaced by the new methods of observation and treatment. Hippocrates himself had noted that the truth of his method was proven by the fact that even the sick who did not believe were helped by it! Unwittingly, he inverted a basic principle of healing practiced in the context of logotherapy.

Another error was the Hippocratics' adherence to the theory of the four humours; blood, phlegm, black and yellow bile bringing disease by their various imbalances. This view limited the possibilities for a rational pathology of specific cause and effect. The Hippocratic pathology, the "dyscrasias" of the four humours, persisted with Galen who willed it to European medicine where it held sway until the eighteenth century. Even Shakespeare, and the layman, Burton, who authored one of the great medical books, The Anatomy of Melancholy, referred regularly to the humours in psychological and physical disease. A third limiting factor in the development of a general pathology among the Hippocratics was their obvious gaps in anatomical knowledge.

Anatomy was not practiced by the members of the Hippocratic school.

Knowledge regarding human function and form was assumed by analogizing from animal dissection and even this was limited until the comparative anatomy of Aristotle. Human dissection, of course, was not regularly conducted until the Alexandrians began post mortem examinations in the first century after Christ, beginning the possibilities for pathologic anatomy which would mature in the seventeenth and eighteenth century.

Hippocrates and his followers maintained other errors. Although familiar with the pulse Hippocrates thought that the pneuma, air or spirit, coursed through the arteries and the liver was the organ of sanguification. Hot blood, "the fire of life," left it by the veins while the heart mixed blood with the pneuma drawn from the lungs by bellows-like auricles. The Hippocratics considered the brain a recepticle for redundant moisture, phlegm, which was discharged to relieve the body of extra heat. They considered the heart the seat of the soul, perhaps explaining Hippocrates' correct observation "that anger contracts the heart and summons heat and fluid to the head while a good frame of mind, euthymie, expands the heart." This suggested possibilities for psychosomatic medicine once the correct orientation of psyche and soma was identified but the depreciation of the verbal mode limited this.

Hippocrates epitomizes the best in Greek medicine with his orientation to natural cause in disease events, the physis, and the emphasis on ecological, social and personal factors. He paid great attention that non-ideological approaches be taken thus both allopathic, contrary cures, and homeopathic, like cures like, approaches were used. He was a bedside doctor, teacher and student. Most importantly, he saw his art as a noble service to the sick. He was never just a scientist but was always careful to conduct his practice with the deep sense of high art the care of the sick demands.

Hippocrates did much but much more wide ranging and significant contributions in philosophy and biology and the methods of scientific study appropriate to living things came with Aristotle. Aristotle is the preeminent figure in Greek natural philosophy. He devoted his life to the observation and investigation of the physical and natural world using the tools of inductive science. He also labored long on the first principles of deductive science which would assist in the acquisition of valid knowledge. He studied under the greatest minds of his age, including Plato, and he tutored the greatest military figure of the ancient world, Alexander of Macedon. He as a man of genius and method whose voluminous writings present a clear legacy: the examination by reason for reason in the sensible world.

Aristotle taught that the world is real in both being and becoming and he showed us a method for gaining new knowledge about it by use of the syllogism, one of Aristotle's great intellectual bequests. It is a primary form of the method of science as it is the method of inference and deduction whereby man adds to his knowledge through reason. Aristotle's great work on knowledge and logic, *The Organon*, includes *The Categories* and *The Analytics*. His work in logic is thought's comment on itself and should be so regarded. *The Analytics* is a commentary on the idea that logic must follow the formal principles of mathematics, reflecting the Pythagorean and Platonic view that the world is knowable through number.

The Analytics hold the key to knowledge. In it Aristotle gives us the premise, the sentence affirming or denying some thing, and the syllogism, "a discourse in which certain things being stated something other than what is stated follows of necessity from their being so."[10] The syllogism assumes that some knowledge is given, i.e., exists, before we undertake the formal exercise of knowing. This knowledge is of what Aristotle calls the "categories." They are both a mental construct and the arrangement of things in material space and include substance, relation, quantity, quality, action, time, place and state. These are a priori; they need not be proven since they are intuitive. They are also confirmed by sense experience and cannot be separated from their real existence in time and place. The syllogism and inferential knowledge have their basis in the categories. Without these there would be no universals on which to build new knowledge through the inference. In contrast, you may recall the philosophy of the Hindu *Carvaka*, which granted ontological status to the world of perception but then denied the validity of inference because it denied the existence of the categories. Later orthodox Hindu systems, on the other hand, accepted the inference but rejected the reality of the world of perception.

There could be no better explanation of Aristotle's method itself than that given in his own words. In *The Topics* he states that reasoning is an argument in which

> certain things being laid down something other than these necessarily comes about through them. It is a demonstration when the premises from which the reasoning starts are true and primary or such that our knowledge of them has originally come through premises which are primary, true. Things are true and primary which are believed on the strength not of anything else but of themselves for in regard to the first principles of science it is improper to ask any further for the why and wherefore of them. Each of the first principles should command belief in and by itself.[11]

The philosophers of modern symbolic logic and logical positivism may have cast this aside in their skeptical refinements, but *a priori* knowledge has been accepted in Western thought since Aristotle.

The *Posterior Analytics* shows that a priori knowledge is indispensible. Speaking about a geometer who was to approach a study of a proof in the triangle, Aristotle points out

> if he, a geometer, did not in an unqualified sense of the term know existence of this triangle, how could he know without qualification that its angles were equal to two right angles? No, clearly he knows not without qualification but only in the sense that he knows universally.[12]

He states that scientific knowledge is a knowledge of causes, the reasons why things are as they are, adding that knowledge also rests on certain premises which are true, primary and independent of demonstration, e.g. causality, change and the fact of existence. Aristotle emphasized the term "physis," and we must understand the term as he meant it. It is customary to translate the Greek "physis" simply as "nature" and to assume Aristotle was therefore studying nature in its material aspects, but he was studying being and physis; being had the all encompassing meaning of "things which exist."

The beginning of Aristotle's treatise on logic sets forth his method with an uncompromising emphasis on the precision of language in the construction of syllogisms and the use of the inference. These constitute both the formal laws of logic and the proper lexical arrangement. It is unarguable that a primary role in his method is accorded to language. One cannot be unmindful of Heidegger's thoughts, on the etymological difficulties inherent in the translation of the Greek through the Latin or through the Syriac and Arabic. "Physis" is the particular root word whose subject is "being" and not merely "nature." From Thales and Parmenides through Plato and Aristotle, the question was one of being and becoming. "Physis," as being, was the original and all determining fact whereas physis, when used to mean nature, is an etymological distortion. Aristotle meant his metaphysics as the study of "being as being" as he himself introduced it. Therefore the study of material being, "physis," through science is the same as the study of being, "physis," in metaphysics. Philosophy, then, makes science because it defines both the reality of the objects of science and the methods by which we know them.

Aristotle taught that material things were composed of matter (substance) and form (their essences, what makes them what they are and not something else) as Plato did. He did not, however, give the forms an independent existence in a world of pure forms. We can make science because we can abstract the formal essence of a thing, its universal characteristic, from its inclusion in particular things. Familiarity with all kinds of trees, for instance, differing in shape, size, or color, allows one to contemplate the idea of the tree, the universal form.

Aristotle's metaphysics connects matter, form, the four causes and the categories, and his logic demonstrates the methods of relating the particulars to the universals. We know the world and develop new knowledge about it because we know things in the world by their form and substance. For Aristotle, as for Plato, science is knowledge of universals, the common principles present in different things but not limited to each particular thing itself. Yet Aristotle disagrees with the Platonic emphasis on a knowledge of pure forms above that of individual things. We can have a mental picture of a tree independent of any existing tree yet it is a picture that all trees would satisfy and Aristotle maintains that there are no pure ideas, of trees, goodness, virtue, or anything else, except as these are in the mind of the first cause (God). Plato had given the pure forms an ideal existence separate both from things and from the divine nous (Demiurgos) and made these the object of scientific knowledge. Aristotle, however, states that we can gain that knowledge solely through the study of everyday things brought to us through the senses and then "known" by an act of the intellect on this information. The important point to note is that Aristotle's position accords with the facts as we, today, have them; scientific knowledge is positive, i.e. demonstrable, knowledge independent of suprasensory or metaphysical categories. Scientific knowledge is knowledge of the "here and now."

Aristotle had a lifelong interest in medicine. His father, Nichomachus, was court physician to Amyntas of Macedon and was a member of the Asclepiads. Aristotle studied at the Academy in Athens with Plato and returned to Macedonia at the request of King Phillip who placed him in charge of the education of his son, Alexander. During the years of Alexander's conquests Aristotle established his own school, the Lyceum, in Athens and remained there until political forces demanded his exile after the death of his benefactor. It has been claimed that his political connections gave Aristotle access to more materials and specimens for study and dissection than would otherwise have ever been possible for a private individual, nonetheless his works form one of the great compendia in the history of nature study.

Aristotle never practiced clinical medicine but he was familiar with the work of Hippocrates and the Pythagoreans, including Alcmaeon, and the works of Empedocles, Democritus and others. Aristotle did not have a theory of the circulation; he taught that the two main vessels, the aorta and vena cava, arose in the heart and went to the head. Others, such as Polybus, the son-in-law of Hippocrates, had erroneously taught that there were four pairs of vessels which went from the head to the heart, one pair traveling down the back of the neck to the hips and then directly down to the feet. A second pair, the jugular vessels, went to the thighs and along the legs to the feet. A third pair went from the head to the internal organs. The fourth pair traveled down the front of the neck to the genitals. This view was shared by Syennesis of Cyprus and Diogenesis of Appollonia.

Apparently Aristotle had distinguished arteries from veins although this had also been credited to Praxagoras of Cos who called the arteries the "air holders." Aristotle, however, is usually cited for naming the aorta, also "air holder," and he assumed that the aorta carried the vital principle. His dissection of the aorta included descriptions of the arteries to the kidneys but he mistakenly made the ureters part of those arteries. He taught that blood traversed the veins into the heart. He thought that the blood and the right side of the heart contained heat and that the heart was the center of intelligence whereas the brain was the organ of cooling, sending phlegm into the heart and blood to moderate their temperature. In principle, then, he agreed with Hippocrates and differed with Alcmaeon who had claimed that the brain was the center of intelligence and the heart the center of emotion.

Aristotle believed that vessels in the extremities and head became so small that their contents discharged as vapor. This was consistent with his teaching that the blood in the veins carried the vital principle from the heart to the head and to the extremities. Aristotle thought that the lungs cooled the body and that the blood vessels to the lungs followed the branches of the trachea receiving air from these tracheal branches and taking it to one side of the heart. This is similar to the Empedoclean idea of pores which transferred air from air vessels to blood vessels.

Aristotle also studied the digestive system and thought that its function was controlled by animal heat, digested food passing with the blood into tiny rootlets. He noted that the epiglottis acted as a valve to keep food in the esophagus and out of the trachea whereas earlier writers had thought that some food passed directly through the trachea into the lungs. Aristotle distinguished the jejunum from the colon and named the rectum (from the word "rectus") as the straight connection from the bowel to the anus. He made the bladder the main reservoir for the vapors from the blood, assigning far less importance to the kidneys, whereas Galen recognized the function of the kidneys, ureter and bladder. Aristotle held that the brain was a bloodless organ, devoid of sensation, and the heart to be the center for all sensate activity. He claimed that the brain did not have any direct connections with the sensory organs even though he had dissected nervous tissue. He obviously confused nerves and blood vessels in his dissections. Curiously, Aristotle commented that under the influence of strong emotions the brain could affect the heart.

Aristotle's study of the homoeomeria, substances formed from the four elements, included flesh, fat, bone and blood. He taught that the blood receives heat from the heart and phlegm from the brain. He commented, as did Plato, that when blood was stirred with a stick, fibers were removed and the liquid which remained did not clot. He apparently noted that blood from animals that had been caught in the hunt tended not to clot as easily as blood taken from animals in captivity. He taught that sperm held the potential to form all the human parts within itself in combination with the formless, passive material provided by the embryo from the female. He thought this formless material was the product of the menstrual cycle. He endorsed the view that all of the human parts were pre-formed but also stated that particular characteristics of each animal species were the last to develop while earlier embryonic life was more plant-like, a hint at the later evolutionary principle of ontogeny.

Aristotle's work in comparative anatomy, physiology, embryology and botany was extensive and original. It is now known that he dissected many species: fowl, pigs, goats, horses, fish, dolphins, apes (including the barbary apes), monkeys, lizards, snakes and other reptiles, and the elephant. His work in comparative anatomy was the most inclusive study of its kind in all of history, a tribute to his thoroughness and his adherence to method, and his work on motion was the background for all subsequent developments in mechanics, the motions of the planets, the physics of falling bodies and ultimately the law of gravity, even though later work refuted his principle of the circular movements of the heavenly bodies, the immutability of the cosmos and his theories on falling bodies. His metaphysics influenced the scholastics. The great schoolmen finally moved through their study of Plato and Aristotle to the idea that the prime mover, the source of all motion and causality, was the personal God of Christianity, though Aristotle probably never held the belief in a personal creator himself.

Aristotle's knowledge was encyclopedic and included study in all the sciences. It is no wonder that his genius and his name would quickly give rise to so many schools of Aristotelianism, beginning with the first interpretations of his work by Andronicus of Rhodes about thirty B.C., a legacy then incorporated into the intellectual and metaphysical systems of two great influences on European history, Islam and Christianity. Islam quickly accepted Aristotle. Christianity accepted Aristotle later, but more decisively in terms of Western science. Aristotle's teaching was brought into the Christian world view primarily through the work of St. Thomas Aquinas, by a great philosophical labor which assured that Aristotelian thought on being, change and reality would be a fundamental treasure of the West and a basis for the development of rational, mature science. So it is that the Middle Ages would not only be a time of theological philosophizing but a time when the Platonic number cosmology and the Aristotelian physis would come to serve the new knowledge of nature which followed.

As we leave the Greeks in our narrative we are reminded that we can never leave them. They were the first Western people to ask scientific questions and to seek scientific answers. True, Greek science was primarily contemplative, as in astronomy, but in biology and in medicine, they began to apply the same kinds of methods that would become standard procedure in laboratory and bedside medicine even in our time. They did not, however, pursue the sciences with the same desire to dominate and control nature as is the case in contemporary Western science. The Greeks, rather, sought to know nature to assist her rather than to change her. Greek medicine, particularly, was reverent of nature and the Hippocratic method at the side of the sick man has always meant watchfulness and expectancy. Likewise the interest in science, including medicine, went hand in hand with the interest in philosophical questions, and Greek scientific knowledge, to the extent we can call it scientific, was always linked to cosmology and philosophy and derived from it. It would be a long time, indeed, before the case would reverse and science would be primary and all philosophical speculations would be derivative. But that takes us to the end of our story, there are others that lie between.

Roman Medicine
The End of the Empire

Rome at the height of empire stretched from the North Sea to North Africa, Spain to Syria, the Elbe to the Euphrates. The Imperial will was fully exercised by the time of Domitian, supervising provincial justice, public works, trade and commerce, tribute and tax. By its third century this empire was near exhaustion. Wars, shortages, unemployment, low productivity and inflation had spent the vitality of the state and resuscitation only postponed its collapse. Emperors were regularly removed by the assassin's hand and poisoner's cup. In the interval between the middle of the second century and the beginning of the fourth century, twenty-six Emperors were murdered. Wars flared on all borders and tribes of "barbari" began their descent. At home half a million shiftless souls roamed the great city, kept alive by the emperor's dole, occupied by his circuses. Throughout the empire bands of desperate men carried on widespread brigandage, peasants were reduced and civil servants coerced into their bureaus. Everywhere the tax collectors appeared, pushed on by the Emperors to practice their skills to the fullest. But the disease had been eating away long before it became terminal.

Diocletian, military dictator after 285 A.D., introduced harsh methods. He rejected the imperial money issue as tax payment and demanded payment in kind. The graineries of the empire received this *annona,* the imperial grain requisition, as tax payment. Land and manpower were the basis of the tax fixed for five year intervals and the coloni and other laborers were tied to the land or to their respective occupations. These finally became hereditary and unnegotiable, by law. In 301 A.D., Diocletian issued his Edict of the

Maximum, fixing prices to halt spiraling costs and ruthless business practices. All foods, all services, all consumer goods were included in this edict. Even lawyers were subject though, not surprisingly, they commanded higher allowances than other professionals. The edict, of course, cautioned against imprudence:

> Since as a guide, fear is always found the most influential preceptor in the performance of duty it is our pleasure that anyone who resists shall for his daring be subject to a capital penalty, nor is he exempt who withdraws from the general market since a penalty should be more severe for him who introduces poverty than for him who harasses it.[1]

So much for the edict. It was despised, violated and unsuccessful. Inflation was not curbed, the currency did not stabilize, and the people did not comply. More was needed and Diocletian obliged by organizing the largest bureaucracy in Rome's history to regiment the entire populace. His secret police, the "Agentes in Rebus" watched all movement, reporting every violator. All the while the Agentes were under the suspicious eye of another agency (correctly known as *Curiosi*). The state presently was everywhere, regulations dictated prices, wage, grain levee, civil service, and, of course, taxes. Money was a daily problem, and with so much bureaucracy and so many seeking to evade it, corruption was rampant. The evidence for the ultimate failure of this totalitarian state was the behavior of Diocletian himself. Continually pressed by his co-regents, he initiated cruel persecutions against the Christians and proceeded with every excess against dissenters. Diocletian finally wearied of all the blood letting and abdicated to his villa in Salona to tend his cabbages and await the scourges of his last illness while the dissolution continued.

The practice of medicine always reflects the moral and ethical tenor of the culture it works in so it comes as no surprise that medicine in the empire was as unworthy as its citizens. There is no record of Roman science and there are no advances in the healing arts other than those brought by the Greeks. With all the military power and administrative genius of the Roman mind, it was still ill-disposed to examine nature and the cosmos scientifically. Imperial Roman civilization was punctuated by indolence, superstition, greed and decadence, so medicine was a dubious and suspect enterprise allowing for all sorts of preposterous methods and remedies.

Roman medicine made little contribution to the employment of rational therapies, orderly approaches to diagnosis and prognosis, or to the separation of the medical art from magic and superstition. It was heavily contaminated by oriental influences beginning with the Etruscan and Eastern mystical rites and magic. The Etruscan influence directed the Roman to such practices as haruspicy and divination by the examination of the entrails and internal organs of animals. The Chaldean astrological method, recall, emphasized divination by observation of the stars, the appearance of comets, eclipses and other extraterrestrial phenomenon. The Romans also borrowed the Oriental and Etruscan interest in chthonic and animal deities and the need to seek out the good will of specific gods for particular medical or civic problems. The Roman religious cults were also healing cults with a heavy dose of folk medicine and superstition.

The Romans were also obsessed with ritual as was continually demonstrated in their medicine. The healing rite had to be precise both in terms of specific utterances, the word charms, and the manipulations performed by the healer. Any mistake in the rite, whether in its verbal or mechanical aspect, demanded that the entire process be repeated. Magic and word charms were used (but without regard to the empirically valid aspects of these methods) delivered in the milieu of the Roman theurgic tendencies. All of this was met with extreme specialization, a tendency in evidence, as we have seen, in many primitive societies.

The Romans practiced incubation, sleeping in the temples of the healing gods in the hopes of cure, a practice inherited from Babylonians, Chaldeans, Egyptians and the Etruscans. The provinces and Rome itself were generously populated with these healing temples. Unlike the case of the Greeks in Asia Minor, Cnidos and Coas, however, where temples diminished as the Greeks advanced rational medicine, the Roman temples continued to provide magical and occult experiences. Many temples had statues of chthonic figures, deities, of sleep and dreams (Oneiros and Hypnos Epidotes) and healing gods. Supplicants left votive offerings, the uterus being the organ most often represented, perhaps because of its power for regeneration and fecundity, and the mysteriousness of the female cycle. The snake was a recurring symbol, the chthonic symbol of death, rebirth, rejuvenation and phallic power.

The Romans adhered to the doctrine of signatures and sympathies. Physical attributes such as color, shape, etc., of plants or organs suggested their appropriateness in specific ailments. The doctrine of sympathies became so base as to suggest that by drinking the blood of a gladiator one might regain strength, or by sleeping with a young man, as Seneca had advised, one would have a return of virility and a reprieve from senesence. The Romans were addicted to methods of divination by haruspicy, astrology and dream interpretation. No good Roman ever made a move without these as a guide to future actions.

Overall, indigenous Roman medicine just never could be identified with medicine as the Greeks understood it, and as the Alexandrians, contemporaries of the empire, were refining and teaching it. In fact, if one accepts the comments of Cato the Censor and Pliny the Elder it would appear that the

Romans did without rational medicine for hundreds of years after Rome's founding. It was left to the incoming Greek and Alexandrian physicians to provide rational approaches. But this Greek influence was not gladly met by proud and sentimental Romans who wished to maintain the purity of the Roman experience, uncontaminated by a low and mendacious art of Greeks.

Greek physicians had been welcomed in the courts and cities of all of the societies of their time. Democedes and Ctesias had served the court of the kings of Persia. Hippocrate's son, Thessalus, served the court of Archelus, one of the successors of Alexander the Great, and Erasistratus, a Greek in Alexandria, served the court of the Ptolemies. In Rome, early on at least, it was another story. Cato continuously riled against medicine and Greek physicians. At the same time he loudly proclaimed the benefits of absurd potions, charms and magic and went on at great lengths about the healing power of cabbage. Cato accused the Greeks of murdering and poisoning and felt their presence further diminished an art he already distrusted. In one of his epistles to his son, Marcus, he had closed with an admonition: "Remember, I forbid physicians for you."

Greek physicians finally established themselves and fared quite well in the practice of medicine in Rome and some of them amassed considerable fortunes, particularly in the service of the emperors. By the time of the Caesars Rome granted citizenship to all physicians, free men or foreigners, and thereafter each emperor had a coterie of physicians and specialists, including herbalists, oculists, magicians, poison experts, lithotomists and dream interpretors. By the time of Constantine physicians were salaried and exempt from compulsory military service or service as decurions (city officials) if they were teachers or chief physicians. Chief physicians, and ex-chief physicians, were exempt from public tax payments and the Theodocian Codes mention that in the Germanic Province at Trier

> chief physicians, knowing their subsistence allowances are paid by the people shall prefer to minister to the poor honorably rather than to serve the rich shamefully...They may also accept those offerings which healthy persons offer for their services but not those offerings of persons in danger of death promise them for saving their lives.

During the time between the end of the republic and the last days of the empire numerous foreign physicians found their way to Rome, to fame, and to fortune. Thessalus came speaking out against medicine and doctors, ridiculing their incompetence and their greed while gaining his own advantage. He became known as "latronikes," Conqueror of Physicians; he should rather have sought the conquest of disease. Andromacus, a Greek, became the physician to Nero at a time when death by poisoning was a reasonable fear. Andromacus was clever enough to introduce theriac, a decoction from vipers and spiders that supposedly neutralized poisons, making a tidy sum for himself pushing his antidote. Symmachus, another Greek, often attended gladiators in their dormatories and patients in their homes with great pomp, accompanied by upwards of a hundred servants and pupils (the first grand rounds?). And one never fails to smile at the wonderfully Latin way of calling things by their right names, as when Argathagus became the first free man to practice medicine, recklessly cutting and cauterizing, killing patients so regularly that he earned the appellation *Carnifex,* "the butcher." Aside from these less esteemable characters, Greeks in residence and Alexandrian physicians did well in Rome; and even a true Roman or two contributed to the history of medicine and to the compilation of facts and materials regarding diagnosis and materia medica.

Cornelius Celsus, whose medical text was the first to be translated in the age of printing, wrote various works on the causes of diseases and on surgical procedures. Celsus was the first to separate the methods of the physician from those of the surgeon. He was Hippocratic in his outlook and in his works expounded the Hippocratic approaches and his own advice about them. He suggested that the arteries contained blood and he provided a description of insanity, then called phrenitis. The most interesting parts of his works, however, were those related to surgery in which he listed his four principles; to add what is defective, to remove redundancies, to unite divided parts and to divide those parts improperly joined. He described methods of amputation, lithotomy, hernia repair, tripining and he wrote extensively on procedures and instruments. He described an extensive pharmocopia, herbal and mineral, available to the Romans of his time. He was the first to record the classic signs of inflammation: calor-heat, rubor-redness, dolor-pain, and tumor-swelling, still learned by every medical student.

Pliny Secundus compiled a list of all the remedies then known. He was reputedly a voracious reader sparing only an hour a day to bathe, and then often dictating to his scribes from his tub. His *Materia Medica* and descriptions of botanical phenomena were, after Aristotle's, the most exhaustive in antiquity. He also reported on medical curiosities and left such descriptions as the one of a young woman known earlier as Aresuca who, while married to a virile young man, slowly developed a beard and other male characteristics whereupon, as Arescon, "he" took a wife. Pliny's greatest moment of intellectual curiosity, however, killed him. Hearing of the goings on in Pompeii he travelled there to record the eruption of Vesuvius and was lost in a lava surge.

The most outstanding names in Roman medicine were non-Roman.

Asclepiades, a Bithynian, practiced according to the principles of Democritus, Epicurus and the atomists. He believed in the theory of the motion of atoms through pores and formulated a corpuscular theory wherein there could be two causes of disease, either through the malfunction of the corpuscles or by a blockage of the pores through which they were to pass in and out of organs. His method was Hippocratic, counseling against overzealous bleeding and purging, and excess in general. He advised that all treatments be undertaken promptly, safely and pleasantly (what happened?). Furthermore, Asclepiades developed a very interesting theory about psychiatric illness. He shared, with Democritus, Leucippus, Epicurus and Lucretius, the notion that the mind included the soul and the sensible attributes, all consisting of spiritualized atoms. He elaborated therefrom a theory of disorder of the brain where the anomalous arrangement of the spiritualized atoms or improper penetration of these atoms contributed to mental illness. His therapies included psychical measures, particularly music and the word charm. His theory of the disease and his treatment suggested an integration of the mind and the senses which was certainly an original contribution for his time.

Dioscorides, a Greek in the service of the army of Nero, wrote an extensive work on materia medica and pharmocoepia (classifying types of remedies and their specific applications). Areteaus, a follower of the Hippocratic school in Rome, was the first to point out that with a cerebral lesion there was paralysis on the opposite side of the body whereas with a spinal lesion the paralysis was on the same side.

Some Alexandrian physicians grouped together as "Methodists," practicing a rigid medicine based on the dogma of humors and strict adherence to regimen. Soranus, Themison, Thessalus, the "Iatronikes," and Asclepiades were Methodists. Their treatments began with a rigorous three day fast, often repeated during the course of a specific treatment. They practiced heavy bleeding and severe application of stimulants and purgatives, heavy sweatings and prolonged baths. Significantly, they counseled that if all else failed the patient should then acknowledge the limits of medicine.

Other Alexandrians, the Pneumatists, were less concerned with therapies but remained occupied with the old question of the life principle (pneuma, spirit). The pneumatist Chrysippus taught that the pneuma resided in the heart, arteries and brain. Areteaus and Archigenes believed the pneuma was non-material and was generated in the heart. Recall that Empedocles and Aristotle had thought that the heart was the center of the "fire of life," but they were obviously unwilling to make a distinction between pneuma, soul, and vital principle. Their view was carried over by the Medievalists who taught that the heart was the center of passions.

In addition to prominent Methodists and Pneumatists Alexandria had been home to many other important physicians. Alexandria was the intellectual seat of the empire in its closing centuries and the roots of its medicine were diverse. Eastern and indigenous influences mixed with Greek scientific medicine, Jewish theurgic medicine and neo-Platonist philosophy. Many came to Alexandria from distant parts of the empire and many passed through her gates on their way to Rome. Soranus, Rufus, Galen, Asclepiades and Dioscorides studied there. Herophilus, one of the first great anatomists, came to Alexandria from Bithynia early in his career. He was the first to dissect the human body with scientific interest. He studied the anatomy and function of the brain and was among the first to distinguish motor from sensory nerves. Erasistratus, a Greek, carried out original work on the brain and circulation. He taught that the pneuma coursed through the arteries but that the vena cava was the great vessel. He believed that the lungs cooled the body and brought the pneuma in through its pores. The most famous physician of them all, however, left Alexandria for Rome.

Galen of Pergamos had an early interest in medicine and intellectual pursuits and soon became thoroughly familiar with the works of Hippocrates and Aristotle, stressing their rational methods, the importance of observation, adherence to logic, the validation of empirical data and the benefits of experiment. He came to Rome from Alexandria in his early thirties and soon distinguished himself as a scholar and clinician. He praised and stressed the harmony and economy of nature while his monotheistic beliefs explained this as issuing from the wisdom of the Creator. The Empedoclean four elements were the basis of his physiology and theory of disease formation. He incorporated the four humors in his therapies, continuously stressed moderation, advising that the physician not harm natural processes but rather direct them to the benefit of his patient. His methods of anatomy and his administration of herbals and medicinals (Galenicals) were considered incontrovertible and practiced to the end of the Renaissance. He separated the diagnostic exercise from prognosis and further separated primary signs, pathognomes, from external signs. He studied the pulse but he did not believe in the circular motion of blood. He did, however, name the phases of the heartbeat and while his anatomy was thorough it was based mainly on studies of the barbary apes.

Galen's anatomical works included the description of the cranial nerves and the distinction between motor and sensory nerves. His theory of the blood had the veins containing the blood and emanating from the liver, while the arteries issued from the heart and contained the pneuma. He related changes in functions to the damage of respective organs and there is no better example of his devotion to detail regarding such changes than his study of the kidneys. He notes that many physicians were continuously denying the obvious facts while rigidly adhering to theory.

> Aesclepiades did this in the case of the kidneys. That these organs are for secreting the urine was the belief not only of Hippocrates, Erasistratus, Praxagoras and all other physicians of emminence, but practically every butcher was aware of this. And the fact that the butcher daily observed both the position of the kidneys and the duct which runs from each kidney to the bladder and from this arrangement infers their characteristic use and faculty is known.

Here Galen could hardly be found guilty of careless observation, his dissections and physiological experiments were models of method and common sense and like the ordinary butcher he would not often lose himself in obscure theory but trusted his own experience, a lesson too frequently forgotten both by the ancients and by the generations of doctors who followed.

One could hardly imagine the corruption in Rome, Alexandria and the rest of the empire in the third and fourth centuries and medicine was not spared in this general dissipation. The streets, temples, public baths and meeting houses were generously populated by charlatans and quacks, ruthless and greedy men. Medicine was quickly falling into the hands of the astrologers, magicians, poisoners, organotherapists and druggers, the latter having developed a vast pharmacopeia, most of it illegitimate and very little of it even occasionally effective. In Alexandria the mix of the cultures and the Eastern influence certainly admitted a more favorable view of magical chemistry, alchemy. Even with the worthlessness of all these remedies there was an awful lot of profit taking throughout the empire. Pliny tells of a physician in Marsailles, Charmis, recieving two hundred thousand sesterce for his cold water prescriptions. Crines in the same area was reputed to be so accurate with his prescriptions and astrology that he amassed a fortune of about twenty million sesterce.

Rome and the cities of the empire housed the archiatri, the public physicians, in abundance. Most of them were freemen and former captives from far lying parts of the empire. They received pay from the state for which they in turn taught their art and treated the poor without charge. Many of the physicians, as Galen himself had done, attended the gladiators and manned the hospitals and medical facilities of the army, the valetudinaria, a forerunner of the great hospitals of the early Middle Ages. Healing and charitable services for the poor and homeless were provided by the Christian communities. With them, however, the emphasis was on the dimension of faith as constituting the most important element in the care of the sick. After

Diocletian's retirement the empire fell further and further into debt and disrepair, and with that, its medicine, its morals, its philosophy withered away.

Chateaubriand caught the "spirit" of the age. Constantine and Maxentius were about to meet at the gates of Rome, and Chateaubriand wrote of that collision:

> The war between two worlds at the Milvian bridge had Maxentius sacrificing lions and opening pregnant women to search the hearts of the unborn for a sign of victory, and consulting all of the pagan books and rituals.

Maxentius symbolized the rot, the illegitimacy and the moral poverty of Roman life. The challenger, Constantine, was to bring a new order.

The Middle Ages

Johann Huizinga introduced his classic, *The Waning of the Middle Ages* with a vivid description of late medieval life:

> All things were of a proud and cruel publicity. Lepers sounded their rattles, beggars exhibited their deformity, every order and state, every rank and profession was distinguished by its costume. Executions and other public acts of justice, hawking, marriages, and funerals were all announced by cryers, processions, songs and music...The lover wore the colors of his lady, companions the emblem of their cofraternity, servants the badges or blazon of their lords. A medieval town did not lose its self in extensive suburbs of factories and villas. Girded by its walls it stood forth as a compact whole, bristling with innumerable turrets. However tall the houses of the noblemen or merchants might be, in the aspect of the town the lofty mass of the churches always remained dominant. One sound rose ceaselessly above the noises of busy life and lifted all things unto a sphere of order and serenity, the bells were in daily life like good spirits which by their voices now called upon the citizens to mourn and now to rejoice, now warn them of danger, now exhorting them to piety.[1]

The Middle Ages is defined by piety but it began with war, the war between the faith and paganism, the paganism of Rome and the heathen paganism of the uncivilized North. Christianity was settling the Germanic tribes and the fragmented empire, preparing the greatest social and ethical rehabilitation in history. Only the moral force and authority of religion had the power to recover the affections of the people within the empire while at the same time civilizing those who lately had assisted its collapse from without. It was a singular undertaking, the erection of a new civilization based on faith and committed to the advancement of the individual and social man because of the imperatives of that faith. Yet this period has been repeatedly characterized as a "Dark Age" by those who failed to see its illuminating force. The Church could not busy itself immediately with the problem of knowledge; it was too busy defining its theology and from this base stabilizing those totally disparate societies, the barbarian and the classical. And she was a dogmatic church, it could not have been otherwise. Her mission was to teach the world, later she could learn from it. Yet conventional secular history ignores the great intellectual effort of the church Fathers and the medieval theologian-philosophers in shaping the climate of thought at that age. There were also immense social needs to be met, food, housing, medical care and education for a vast, untamed land—the West.

Thinking about Science was a luxury the nascent West could not yet afford; mind and spirit were needed to spread the faith and tend to the prodigious practical work at hand. Nonetheless, science would become a part of Western civilization because of the Church's belief that all knowledge is good. Knowledge further reveals the majesty and order of creation and helps men to better meet their obligation to the social gospel.

The acceptance of the natural order as good, useful and knowable was in evidence with the early Fathers for as they taught and preached they were confronted by the various heresies which took a dim view of the real world, picturing it as improbable, chaotic, and evil. The Fathers met the heresies head on. The world, they said, is neither illusory nor unknowable, and when there is evil it is man's task to bring good. The heresies, you see, posed an immediate practical danger; by devaluing the world they minimized the need for action directed to social justice or thinking directed to positive knowledge. Arianism, Gnosticism, Nestorianism and Manicheanism were heavily weighed down with the negating spirit of the east with all that implied, including the futility of the ideas and methods of science.

The Christian community, on the other hand, was open to science because it was open to all of the possibilities of the "real" world. Many Churchmen were physicians concerned with practical results gained through the medical art for the practice of the social gospel as well as with the relation of medicine to the growth of knowledge. Tertullian called medicine the sister of philosophy. He was acquainted with Stoic and Sicilian medicine and wrote extensively on medical subjects. Orabasius of Pergamon compiled all of the medical works of his time and Alexander of Tralles studied the nervous system and mental disease. Paul of Aegina wrote on lithotomy, hernia repair and various surgical cures. Eusebius, author of "The Ecclesiastical histories" was influential in the development of public hospitals and hospices, an enterprise which the early Church undertook with vigor. Many others were involved with empirical medicine because it was a necessary part of their secular mission and if this medicine wasn't mature science neither was it ignorance.

The most illustrious figure in the Church early in its development was Augustine of Hippo. Augustine's theology had evolved after flirtations with Arianism and Manicheanism and Greek speculative thought. His philosophy was a blend of Neo-Platonic metaphysics, Christian revelation, and an interest in nature and natural philosophy. He was familiar with biology, medicine and scientific writings of his time and was one of the first to comment that the brain contained three ventricles: the anterior brain for feeling and emotion, the posterior part of the brain for motion, and a third part, above the other two, for memory. He knew the relationship between the nerves and the spinal cord and thought arteries were air passages because they were empty after death. In *De Civitas Dei* he described dropsy, tuberculosis, elephantiasis, and gout, noting that the gout could arise from intemperance or poor heredity. He collected medical anecdotes and in his *De Anima* he mentions the story of a friend, Anicus, who was a professor of rhetoric at Carthage. Apparently, the unlucky Anicus had lost an eye and later begot a son with only one eye. Augustine thought that the two misfortunes were biologically related.

Augustine believed in the beauty and rationality of creation and did not accept the Manichean or even the Platonic view of the natural realm. He rather anticipated the medievalists who joined natural philosophy to their theology. "The world in its orderly series of changes," he wrote, "its mobility, bears witness that it was made by One, invisible and mighty Who is expressed to man in time and space,"[2] those two entities of the Newtonian cosmos derived from the Aristotelian idea of final and efficient cause.

One of Augustine's great contributions was the affirmation of the principle of direct creation. The Neo-platonist thinkers Plotinus, Porphyry and Proclus had taught the idea of emanationism—all existing things overflowing from God as light diffuses from the sun. The primary emanation is nous, the world soul, from which individual souls and forces are ultimately derived which guide and produce matter. The Neo-platonists used the series of emanations to argue that matter in the world of things is imperfect, because of its remoteness from the One. This notion, of course, implies the world is something less than is presumed by the principle of direct creation.

Augustine rejected Neo-platonic emanationism and taught that God created the world "ex-nihilo," by an act of His will and love, and that He created it rationally. The concept of direct creation defined a fundamental difference between Christianity and Eastern and Platonic thought. Augustine did something more, however. He asserted that man can acquire positive knowledge because he can be certain that he thinks, a point that Descartes asserted in the seventeenth century both in his method and as a proof of God's existence. Augustine, therefore, even with his essentially Neo-platonist-Christian synthesis indirectly moved Christian thought toward the validation of sense experience and to knowledge of existing things, a concept fully developed by St. Thomas.

The political character of the early church, in the meanwhile, took shape as the Roman state fell into a condition of political inertia after the emperors moved out and the Franks moved in. The Church introduced the only principal whereby any temporal power could endure: the natural law demand of obedience to the sovereign. At the same time She adopted the model of Roman administration while providing the only alternative to the moribund state. In the fifth century The Merovingian King of the Franco-Germanic nations, Clovis, accepted Christianity on the insistence of his wife Clothilda. Clovis was the first "European" political figure, unifying the German nations under Christianity. Clovis was followed by the Carolinigians and Pepin the Short, the son of Charles Martel, the hero of Tours. Pepin's son, Charles, inherited his kingdoms and moved to consolidate his power while the Bishop of Rome sought the protection of the Frankish chief to offset the threats to the Church from the East. On Christmas day, 800, Pope Leo crowned Charles the Holy Roman Emperor and a new era began.

The alliance between the Church and Charles was of primary importance in the development of Europe. Charles protected the Church and the West from the intense military and social pressure of Islam, allowing the Church to continue its mission of conversion and education.

Charlemagne created the medieval school system. He established cathedral and monastic schools under church supervision directed to the instruction of the monks, community leaders, bishops and members of the court. Teachers came from Ireland and England and established monasteries throughout Western Europe. These monks were an important factor in the civilizing process. They visited all of the Germanic nations, opening centers of learning, transmitting an oral tradition, performing tedious and voluminous manuscript work, maintaining the continuity of philosophical thought inherited from antiquity. Charlemagne encouraged this and was influential in founding a school at Tours and the first schools of the University of Paris which would later become the greatest university of the Middle Ages. Under the auspices of churchmen such as Boethius, Cassiodorus, the Venerable Bede and others, the classical learning was preserved and translated. Charlemagne's Age did not produce any advances in knowledge but the classics were used for secular and clerical instruction, and with great clerics such as

Alcuin of York as the teachers, for the next two centuries churchmen spread the classical learning.

The Church was not the only force in Europe at this time, however. Islam was a powerful counter to the message and methods of Christianity, but Islam also brought the Arabic translations of the classics, more voluminous and complete than those that had been carried out in the West. The Arabs translated the Greek masters and made them available for translation into Latin in the West. The Arabs emphasized Aristotelian physics: motion, quantity, velocity, time, and Aristotelian biology and nature studies, incorporating parts of this into the Kalam, the book of Islamic natural theology. Translations of Aristotle had begun earlier. Andronicus of Rhodes had completed his commentaries on Aristotle's work thirty years before Christ and Boethius had translated the *Physics* and the *Prior* and *Posterior Analytics* in the fourth century. The bulk of the Aristotelian corpus, however, was handed down by the philosopher-physicians of the Islamic culture who also drew on Alexandrian philosophy and science and Jewish metaphysics and theurgic medicine.

Rhazes, the first great figure in Arabian science, was a Persian physician who studied at Baghdad in the early tenth century. He wrote over 200 books in the natural sciences emphasizing the infectious diseases, including small pox which he distinguished from measles. He encouraged evaluation of patient at the bedside and application of Hippocratic treatments. Ibin Sina (Avincenna), another Persian, wrote *The Canon,* a synthesis of the medicine of Galen and Hippocrates and the biology of Aristotle. *The Canon* included extensive discussions of drugs, diseases, methods of treatment, hygiene and public works and was one of the major compendia through which the works of the masters were transmitted to the European world. Albucasis of Cordova wrote a general surgical treatise which revealed the Arabian skill in surgery, limited only by the religious ban on anatomizing. Avenzoar and Averroes were eminent physician-philosophers who made substantial contributions to the literature of medicine, surgery and pharmacy. Maimonides of Cordova, a Jewish pupil of Averroes, was the philosopher-physician to the sultan of Cordova. He wrote on diet, regimen, and the classic *The Causes of Symptoms* in which he elaborated the various factors in disease including the psychological. Maimonides noted that "concern and care should always be given to the movements of the psyche. These should be kept in balance, in the state of health as well as in disease."[3] He recognized the importance of emotions in physical illness and tried to form this into a basic principle of therapy.

Arabian medicine emphasized chemical and herbal remedies; the Arabs brought many of the exotic herbal cures from the Orient and introduced Alexandrian and Oriental alchemical practices. The Arabs also established medical schools in their centers of culture and the first medical school, Gondishapur, dates back to the fifth century although it was formally established by Al Mansoor in the eighth century. Cordova became the leading medical school in Moorish Spain in the eleventh and twelfth centuries and the schools in Baghdad, Fez, and Damascus were important Eastern centers.

Arabian medicine and astronomy borrowed heavily from the Greek and Alexandrian authorities, as did Arabian philosophy. The lack of additions to the heritage of Greek science made by the Arabs was due primarily to the constraint placed on Arabian natural philosophy by its theology. This theology emphasized the direct intervention of God in the cosmos without His natural laws which, in effect, were the intermediate causalities Western science later sought to understand. Certainly, the Islamic belief in a God Who creates and superintends each person and thing, directly, completely dominated the philosophical, cultural and scientific pursuits of Islamic culture and perhaps, thereby, retarded them. Some Islamic contributions in natural philosophy were original but many of these reveal intellectual indebtedness to the Greeks and the Persians. The Arabs saw Aristotle as the master but credited the Persians for original scientific knowledge, a theory of logic and natural science prior to the Greeks. Nonetheless, the Aristotelian corpus formed the basis of the Islamic possibilities in the natural sciences.

Ibn Khaldun, in his great philosophical and sociological introduction to history, *The Muquaddimah,* discussed the various kinds of sciences recognized by the Arabs. He lists the science of logic as the mother science:

> God created in man the ability to think, through it he perceives the sciences and crafts...Knowledge is either a perception of the essence of things or it is apperception, that is, a judgement that a thing is so. Man's effort to obtain knowledge desired requires discernment so that he can distinguish between right and wrong. This process became the canon of logic.[4]

Ibn Khaldun states that Aristotle was the father and systematizer. "He assigned to logic its proper place as the first philosophical discipline and the introduction to philosophy, therefore he is called the first teacher." Khaldun listed physics, the study of natural sciences, medicine, agriculture and metaphysics as the main sciences of man. His discussions of sorcery, alchemy, talismans, the science of letters and magic words distinguished the usefulness of these when God, Allah, was invoked, from their debasement when pursued in their own right. In the *Muqaddimah* God dictates all human behavior and is the source of all wisdom and knowledge. He alone is the object of all man's efforts in philosophy and science. It is not necessary to study the cosmos and nature so much as it is to know the Maker directly.

The Kalam, the philosophy of Islam, developed alongside the rigid exegesis of the Koran. The Kalam, however, saw nature from the perspective of the Greek physical and metaphysical tradition, including Pre-Socratic atomism. The Kalam taught atomism through God's creative acts and what it termed "the three meetings" of scripture with philosophy. The first was with Philo and his followers at Alexandria, the second with the fathers of the early Christian church, and the third meeting was with the Mutakallimun, the interpreters of Islamic philosophy and religion. The Mutakallimun accepted atomism because it was consistent with their idea of direct creation of the world and all matter without intermediate causality. Thus, their view differed both from Aristotle's which held that the cosmos is timeless and uncreated and the Neo-platonist tradition of emanationism. The Greeks, at least Aristotle and Plato, and the early Christian fathers taught a species of atomism but believed that God acted through the intermediate agency of causality. Democritus and his followers had preached the theory that bodies consist of infinite numbers of atoms existing from eternity prior to their formation into material being by God. The Kalam accepted this while rejecting intermediate causality because that seemed to place limits on God's creative act. Of course, the denial of contingency and levels of causality limited the possibilities for natural science since it made the study of causality and natural laws superfluous. The knowledge of God is all inclusive and He is the only cause man should study.

Arab culture diminished as it came under increasing assault from the Turks and the Mongols, while the Crusades in the West forced a withdrawal from Spain, the last and most glorious Islamic foothold in Europe. Arabic grandeur in Sicily had already been replaced by the Norman presence under Roger II and then by the Hohenstaufen under Frederick II, so that Islam was steadily repairing to its origins in the East. At the same time the expansion of Christian Europe continued and much of that expansion was the result of the rise of the universities whose foundations were built by the Church.

The first university in the West which could claim the name was established in Salerno in Southern Italy. It was renowned for its medical school and the teaching of the Hippocratic and Galenic doctrines. Salerno, however, was eclipsed by Montpelier, famous for its medicine and Bologna, the center for Canon and Roman law. But the greatest of the medieval universities was at Paris, started as the cathedral school of Notre Dame. It was a thriving intellectual community in the middle of the twelfth century and the center for much of the philosophical encouragement for the interest in natural science.

Paris and environs had been particularly fertile ground for learning. The school of Chartres, outside of Paris, and the school of St. Victor on the west bank of the Seine were early centers of learning. The school of Chartres was Aristotelian but studied Plato's metaphysics in the *Timaeus* and started the synthesis of the Aristotelian and Platonic philosophies under Abelard of

Bath, Bernard, and John of Salisbury. The school of St. Victor taught Platonic philosophy through the works of St. Augustine. At the university, however, the real Aristotelian "Regiornomento" began.

William of Auvergne was the first interpreter of Aristotle at Paris, and he was followed by Robert Grossotesta who influenced Roger Bacon, Albert Von Bollstaed (Albert the Great) and Thomas Aquinas. Albert was the leading Aristotelian at the University of Paris in the early thirteenth century and the preeminent figure in natural science in medieval Europe. Among his pupils Thomas stood out as a gifted intellect and promising heir to Albert's work in Aristotelian philosophy. They moved to Cologne where Albert established a school based on the Lyceum, teaching much of what Avicenna had taught while adding elements of Neo-platonism, improving the synthesis which aided medieval scientific thought. It remained for Thomas to perfect that synthesis and to incorporate Aristotle decisively into Catholic theology.

Thomas was the greatest mind of the age. He accomplished a philosophical synthesis of Aristotle and Plato while modifying both and working this into the structure of belief. At the same time, Thomas was able to draw the best from Arabian and Jewish treatments without prejudice. Thomas emphasized the goodness, usefulness and rationality of creation. He asserted the regularity, order and symmetry of the natural world, and he affirmed the reality of "physis" as the basis for scientific knowledge. This was an extremely important point, and one which was too often forgotten in subsequent philosophical debates, down to our time. Thomistic philosophy had important implications for science because of some of its first principles. Thomas taught that being is real and is realized in particular things, and that scientific knowledge derives from our knowledge of particular things first gained through sense experience. This knowledge (cognition) results from the mental process of abstracting concepts. Thomas emphasized that the goal of cognition is the knowledge of things in themselves and not simply a knowledge of our own ideas (concepts). In this sense Thomas is a realist rather than an idealist and the point is especially important as it is clear that if the goal of cognition were the concepts we formed rather than the things we are studying then a science of real things would not be possible. Thomas' realistic philosophy and psychology, then, serves as a basis for valid science in their emphasis on the reality of existing things and the certainty of our knowledge about them.

Note should be made here of the relation between Thomas' realism and the views of a fourteenth century Franciscan, William of Ockham, often considered an important figure on the road to science. Ockham taught a type of Nominalism which suggested that forms, universals, have no real existence in things themselves but are mental constructs. These forms are not referrable either to objects or to any "ideas" in the mind of God. Ockham's Nominalism or Terminism (universals are terms or natural signs) has been interpreted as a new direction toward positive knowledge. St. Thomas, however, taught that science is knowledge of universals; he differed from Ockham only in where he placed the universals. In that regard Ockham cannot be said to represent an advance over Thomas since they both recognized that the validity of science rests in raising it from the particular to the universals. On the other hand, one could argue that Ockham's view is more congenial to the scientific method in so far as his universals were independent of ideas in the mind of God. To this extent this is meant to undervalue the Thomastic understanding of science, however, the distinction is useless.

Thomas never felt that his realistic philosophy would subvert either revelation or science and he believed that scientific study would support the theological propositions regarding cosmos and nature. He also felt that Aristotle's philosophy of knowledge and his scientific methods reflected this same emphasis on the reality of existing things. Thomas was not an experimental scientist and he did not make any specific contribution in natural philosophy; rather his general understanding of the methods and possibilities knowledge including that specific kind of factual knowledge we call scientific, was a theological affirmation. For Thomas, the Christian and the scientist could be the same man.

Thomas was a theologian, his mission was the truth of Christianity which he saw as an all encompassing statement about God's creation; cosmos, nature and rational man. The Christian, Thomas said, must believe, but he must also use reason to know as best he can the most that he can, for it would be a frustration of the Divine plan to possess reason only to neglect it in the search for the truth. With the faculty of reason man can know that God exists, he can know his own existence and that of all existing things and he can develop positive, i.e. scientific, knowledge because of these.

Significantly, much of Thomas's efforts on behalf of reason and faith were directed toward fellow Christians, philosophers such as Siger of Brabant who had interpreted Aristotle's emphasis on reason and the reality of existing things more radically. These followers of Averroes had moved to a denial of personal immortality and the special creation of the natural order. Thomas saved his best intellectual rebuttals for them, assuring them that the Catholic interpretations of Aristotle would reject such radical editing while bringing Aristotelian thought into harmony with traditional church teaching. Ironically, Thomas was attacked by the conservatives for his own radicalism, the incorporation of the "pagan" Aristotle into his "Summa" so that in 1277 the Bishop of Paris, Tempier, placed the works of Thomas on the index, along with those of Siger. Thus, the first reception of the *Summa Theologica* was an official condemnation, though not a Papal one.

Thomas had prepared well for his work. He had studied with the Dominicans and then in Paris with Peter of Ireland, a great Aristotelian. He met Albert, travelled with him to Cologne where he was ordained, and returned to Paris to continue his own work with William of Moerbeke, a Greek specialist who translated Aristotle for him. Thomas drew heavily from *The Physics* and *De Anima* of Aristotle in assisting the development of medieval science. In the *Physics* Aristotle had discussed matter, form, causality and place and time. He taught that motion was related to all of these, issuing from a first cause which the Christians understood to be the Creator. Albertus (Magnus) and Aquinas both recognized that Aristotle's motion (change) was an inherent property of all material things. This potency or entelechy was a property of being itself. Matter contains within itself the possibility of becoming something else in so far as all things are composed of prime matter which is pure potency. This is in addition to the fact that prime matter gives things their accidental properties in relation to pure form, which makes them what they are. Much of this is a restatement of Aristotle, clarified and amplified by St. Thomas. Thomas also refined Aristotle's thoughts on time and change. Aristotle had defined time as the measure of motion (change) but he had wondered whether or not the measurement was a product of contemplation or was real in itself. Both Aquinas and Magnus taught that time and the other categories were real, independent of the activity of the mind.

Thomas was a realist. He said that nothing is known in the mind which is not first perceived by the senses, a principle underlying all of Thomas' natural philosophy, making the objective world of matter and form independent of the perceiving being. Thomas perfected Aristotle by teaching that material beings are composed of matter and form which exist together and cannot be considered apart. Nature, as matter and form, reflects God's plan and reveals His rational, creative and sustaining impulse in all existing things. This was consistent with the medieval view of beauty which, as Huizinga pointed out, was the idea of "perfection, proportion and splendor." The world is good and was to be studied as good because the Creator is good. The reason for making science is to know the Maker! Thomas offered a philosophy which was congenial to natural science and taken in its unity, his theology, philosophy and "common sense" view of the world were the most internally consistent to issue from the pens of the many original and profound thinkers of the period.

The Dominicans, Vincent of Beauvais, Albert and Thomas himself, worked in Paris using translations of Aristotle by James of Venice and Gerard of Cremona, and the sixth century translations by Boethius as well as those of

William of Moerbeke. At the same time a group of Franciscans was working at Oxford studying Aristotle and natural philosophy. The great figures in this Oxford movement were Robert Grossetesta, formerly at Paris, later Bishop of Lincoln and Chancellor of Oxford, and Roger Bacon, one of the fathers of the inductive method and empirical chemistry. Bacon had originally studied in Paris with Grossetesta and the Dominican Robert Kilwardby, who became Archbishop of Canterbury and an Oxford professor. Kilwardby had stated that qualities in phenomena are in bodies themselves and are not products of the mind, the very point made by Thomas. Kilwardby also emphasized the importance of mathematics in relation to natural philosophy. Bacon and Grossetesta continued Kilwardby's thinking in the thirteenth century and became the most famous of the Oxford Aristotelians. All three taught the mathematical structure of the cosmos and nature, and they cited as evidence the importance of mathematics in astronomy and optics. They emphasized the Platonic and Pythagorean idea that precise knowledge is mathematical. At the same time they were committed to the Aristotelian economy by virtue of its emphasis on rational demonstration, method and observation. Bacon himself had claimed that observation and experiment made for the correctness and exactness of science while mathematics was its measure.

The Oxford philosophers were not alone in crediting mathematics with importance for the development of valid science. Albert had said that mathematics was a high science derived from the categories that make up nature itself, the mental abstraction that man performs in describing reality and Bacon and Grossetesta, while teaching the Aristotelian method and observation which is particularly useful in the biological sciences, still regarded mathematics as the mode for study of the physical world.

The Oxford tradition continued with Thomas Bradwardine, another Archbishop of Canterbury. Bradwardine was one of the great scientific minds of his time, perhaps the leading scientific mind in England in the fourteenth century. His works included treatises on proportions of velocities in moving bodies and a mathematical law of dynamics which anticipated Newton's. He taught that motion was a principle of velocity, a ratio of distance to time rather than an Aristotelian function of potency. This was a very advanced idea, one which was to become a cornerstone of the physics of Galileo and Newton.

The distinguished lineage of theologians who were natural philosophers in the thirteenth and fourteenth centuries brought Aristotelian physics and scientific philosophy into the substance of university teaching while the characteristically Western interest in the development of scientific and mathematical principles in describing physical events gradually began to take hold. The impetus for this was theological, the belief in the rational order of nature and physical events and the importance of applying human reason to discovery of the Creators' laws in nature. This interest in natural philosophy began with the schoolmen, Albert and Thomas, and continued with the mathematical philosophers of Oxford, only some of the important ones cited here. Their names, however, are not so important as their ideas which prepared the way for the advances in physics and cosmological studies culminating with Newton and the displacement of Aristotelian physics by Newton's kinetics. This new mathematical physics had its roots in the medieval interest in the idea of science and its importance in the acquisition of new knowledge.

Physical science was not the only science which was advancing gradually in the late Middle Ages and the Renaissance. Medicine was also developing through a similar evolution and acceptance of scientific methods. In the Middle Ages medicine was an activity of the Church rather than a profession and it was hardly scientific in its every day application. The Church was working in a part of a world that had been tribal and this had a great bearing on the practical conduct of medicine. The Churchmen, monks and preachers relied on the Greek medical tradition and the folk medicine proper to the Teutonic-Celtic peoples with its abundance of magic and priestly healing. The Druids, like the Pythagoreans, were involved in mystical language, numerology and cult healing, word charms, music, herbals and minerals. Magic scripts such as the Runic of the northern Teutons and the Ogham of the Celts formed the basis for a mystical language culture. The medical practices of the Teutonic-Celts used this word magic and spiritualism in striking contrast to the developing scientific medicine of the universities.

The scientific medicine that was introduced into Europe came, in part, by way of Islamic contacts in Syria, Constantinople, Sicily and Spain and was Greek medicine in its origins. In these centers there was a cultural exchange in philosophy, natural science and medicine. The Arab proclivities for magical chemistry, alchemy and herbal and mineral remedies joined evolving Western medicine, especially in Spain and Southern Italy. The school at Salerno, already an important medical center in the ninth century, was the first Western institution to systemize all of these converging doctrines and heritages. At Salerno Christians, Arabs and Jews studied the works of Hippocrates and Galen and the classical foundation for medical teaching in Europe. Salerno was the first lay center for medical teaching and practice in which a formulary of herbals and minerals and a materia medica were developed and used in practical treatment. Animal dissection was practiced with scientific methodology and the customary and traditional healing methods were recorded in a famous Salernitan poem on regimen, diet and Hippocratic method. Here, too, surgery was conducted with more advanced techniques than elsewhere. A famous text by Roger of Salerno described rectal and gynecological operations and operations for hernia, kidney stones and orthopedic repairs. The University at Montpelier was the immediate successor to Salerno and numbered Arnold of Villanova, Raymond Lull, John of Arderne and Guy de Chauliac among its elite. Arderne became the most famous English surgeon of the fourteenth century while de Chauliac enjoyed the same status in France. Both stressed the importance of anatomy for surgery and careful operative techniques along with the judicious application of their art in the assistance of nature.

Italy was the home of the two most famous medical schools of the age, Bologna and Padua. Both centers introduced the case report, clinical case descriptions gathered from observations at the bedside. The first anatomical theatre was built in Padua in the middle of the fifteenth century though dissection had been practiced there for at least a hundred years. The first clinical autopsy was conducted in the latter part of the thirteenth century at Bologna, the home of Mondino, the first great anatomist after Galen. The stimulating investigative atmosphere at these Italian centers and at the Papal medical School in Rome was a primary factor in the development of scientific anatomy, physiology and clinical medicine in the centuries that followed. At the same time, particularly in southern Italy and Sicily, physicians were first regulated by the state.

Frederick II was the first European monarch to license physicians in Naples and Roger of Sicily required a state examination at Palermo. This court interest in medicine paralleled a Papal concern for the legitimacy of medical and surgical methods. It was common, therefore, for secular figures, Pope or high clerics, and physicians to assist each other both regarding practical medical problems and the advancement of medical learning. The Church was congenial to these efforts and encouraged scientific medicine while the interaction between secular and church figures was an incentive to the scientists. Astronomers, physicians and chemists could find benefactors in the church or court and in turn would serve the papacy or the crown, practicing their specialities or providing teaching and consultation. The Popes, especially, had an ongoing interest in science and were attended by the leading physicians and astronomers. The Papacy supported the advancement of science without seeing this as an effort that could prejudice the revealed word.

The growing interest in natural philosophy and legitimate science in the later Middle Ages is an unarguable fact. The teachings of Grossetesta, Bacon and Marsh in Oxford and Aquinas and Magnus in Paris lent great impetus to the idea that science had a practical aim and a theological basis which were concordant. Dawson made the distinction between this development in the West in the Middle Ages and scientific interests among the Greeks and the Arabs. He notes that Greek science was "essentially intellectualist, it was the contemplation of reality as an intelligible order." The Greeks were less interested in practical results; besides some advances in astronomy, mechanics and medicine, Greek science never realized its earlier promise and remained theoretical. Islamic science, on the other hand, was basically magical as evidenced by the interest in alchemy and magical chemistry even if this foreshadowed developments in scientific chemistry. The Arabs viewed any contradictions to religious teaching with intense skepticism, thus an emphasis on natural philosophy and science for its own sake was far less important to them. Dawson notes that Arabian scientists sought "not knowledge but power to discover the elixir of life, the philosopher's stone. Astronomy was inseparable from astrology and chemistry from alchemy. In a word, Arabic science was magic."

In the West, however, science was regarded as having increasing importance even though the great number of scientists still mixed their astronomy with astrology, their medicine with occult healing and their physics with Neo-platonic mysticism. Yet, these men helped to develop an attitude more appropriate to the careful observer than to the occult magician. The universities also aided in the development of the new knowledge and gradually eroded the position of the clergy and monks in the delivery of medical care, making this an increasingly lay function. They fostered a concern for anatomical and surgical principles and rational treatment methods, and they were supported by the Popes, particularly in the universities in Italy. The Medieval universities presented medicine, astronomy and all of the other natural sciences within the context of Christian philosophy. Virtually all of the great minds of the age worked within that framework, a philosophical structure that informed all of science until the modern era.

Outside of the universities, different conditions prevailed, at least with regards to medicine. While the great masses of people still had their faith, that appeared to be all they had. The practical conduct of medical care and healing was in the hands of untrained women, folk healers and clerics. Few healers and physicians were licensed, fewer still had ever witnessed an anatomy session and almost all were ignorant of the classical medical works. A distinction between physicians and surgeons was made and the surgeons increasingly suffered ridicule since barbers still performed blood-letting and minor operations. The surgeons were distinguished by their ignorance of Latin, their non-standing in the universities, and the final ignominy, their poverty. Some recovered nicely as journeymen lithotomists and herniotomists, travelling from town to town caring for the farmers, peasants and poor in great numbers.

A legion of quack nostrums and bizzare remedies saw their way into healing, as they always have. Yet many of the folk cures were empirically valid. Herbal and chemical treatments, of course, were popular, perhaps more so at this time than previously because of the Arabian influences. The alchemy of Alexandria, brought to Europe by the Arabs, was the most interesting of the "arts" in the Middle Ages. Alchemy was a blend of rigid methodology and occult magic combined to produce the transmutation of metals and the production of gold. The details of such transmutation were hidden so that alchemists became more akin to members of secret sects, initiates into sacred mysteries. With the growing interest in natural sciences, however, and a renewed emphasis on careful observation and experiment, alchemy gradually took on the form of scientific chemistry

The best minds since the era of the pre-Socratics had been involved in theories about the constitution of matter and the transformation of elements and metals. Early minerology and Hindu and Egyptian herbal and chemical practices passed through Alexandria and were delivered by the Arabs to the West. Leading intellectuals in the West including the Oxford scholars, Grossetesta and Bacon, Albertus in Paris and Vincent Beauvais and Arnold deVillanova either experimented alchemically or wrote about such methods. Roger Bacon was certainly one of the most active alchemists of his age, and his experiments with transmutation are a mix of occult and scientific methods. He was familiar with the production of gunpowder and described the explosive properties of various mixtures of saltpeter, sulphur and charcoal. He subscribed to the ancient idea of the generation of materials and minerals from primary elements and he worked on the formation of colors and the refinement of medicinals but in these activities Bacon also employed methods which made him a leader in the science of the day. In the fourteenth century, the Benedictine, Basil Valentine, also performed chemical experiments. He introduced antimony into medical treatment and reportedly described the chemical process for making muriatic acid and he was a leading figure in the early development of the chemical sciences as applied to medicine. More famous than either Valentine or Bacon, however, was the alchemist-physician, Paracelsus.

Paracelsus Theophrastus vonHonhenheim was one of the most interesting and enigmatic figures of his time bridging, as he did, the medieval and Renaissance worlds. He was born in Einsiedlen in Switzerland in 1493. He studied medicine and alchemy in Vienna and Italy and graduated medicine at Ferrara in 1530. He travelled throughout Europe and visited the leading universities. All the while his interest in medicine grew. He viewed his practice of medicine as a "sacred task, a kind of priestly mediation between God and patient." His theological urges involved him in occult and magical pursuits. He studied astrology in an effort to explicate the meaning of man and his interaction with the cosmos, and alchemy to explore symbolically his psychic transformation. Paracelsus travelled to Basel in 1427 and quickly won fame after healing some of its prominent citizens. He spoke out against the hypocrites in medicine and public life, assuring a quick dismissal from Basel and a journeyman's career. He became increasingly philosophical but continued to see large numbers of patients, especially among the poor whose ranks he had entered. He died at an inn in Salzberg after delivering his will in September of 1541.

Paracelsus built his medicine on a knowledge of astronomy, alchemy, philosophy and ethics and the methods of observation and experiment. He understood disease and healing in their spiritual aspects. He anticipated psychotherapy with insights he gained from his keen interest in men as men and not merely as medical cases. He strongly believed in the power of the curing word, the magical symbolism of alchemy and the notion of diseases as related to man's fallen condition. Yet he saw the majesty of his fellow man as the center and focus of being and knowledge. "The whole world surrounds man as the circle surrounds the point. Wisdom can be achieved only through the attractive force of the center and the circle." He was interested in improving the standards of the physicians. He advised that "it must not surprise the physician that nature is more than his art for what can equal the forces of nature. He who has no expert knowledge of them has not mastered the art of medicine." He did not fail to see the danger of abstract knowledge. "Every physician must be rich in knowledge and not only that in books. His patients should be his book, no one can learn his trade from books but only from experience, theory and practice should remain undivided!"[10]

Paracelsus understood that the physician's responsibility was, as Hippocrates had counseled, to "do no harm." He advised a life of study coupled with preceptorships with wise teachers. But he also respected the experience of old fools, "...the physician does not learn everything at high colleges. From time to time he must consult old women, gypsies, magicians and peasant folk."[11] How right he was! The eradication of small pox began after Edward Jenner listened to a dairy maid of Gloucestershire tell how she could not possibly contract the pox because she had suffered the cow pox. Likewise, the most popular heart pill, digitalis, came after William Withering saw Shropshire peasants using foxglove for dropsy. Nor did Paracelsus fail to see that there were men of low nobility in medicine, "So great is the ill will among some physicians that each denies honor and praise to the other. They would rather harm a patient than grant a colleague his meed of praise."[12]

Paracelsus was a representative figure in a time of transition as his life and work illustrate the mix of science and mystery, the urge, on the one hand, to break from tradition and dogma by experiment and the tendency to drift back into magical methods and spiritual thinking. Certainly the late Middle Ages was a period in which the scientific impulse mixed with magic and ritual in alchemy, in astrology, and in the healing arts. The Middle Ages, of course, allowed for a belief in ghosts, demons, witches and for belief in God, angels and benevolent spirits and Medieval cosmology and natural philosophy reflected this. The Ptolemaic astronomy still held sway and its geocentricity was concordant with the Christian view that man, though fallen and base, is still the centerpiece of biblical creation. Medieval chemistry, as well, did not limit itself to empirical method, but employed spiritual forces, secret and mysterious formulae and recitations, and the belief in transmutation itself. Likewise, the physician or healer could not ignore the effects of spirits, good or bad, nor fail to incorporate his religious faith into the healing rituals and practices.

The end of the Middle Ages, then, was not a single event. Just as the opening of the Middle Ages was no age of darkness, so its closing was not a sudden leap into Renaissance enlightenment, for at both ends the occult mixed with the rational as was so well exemplified by Paracelsus. The Middle Ages gave Western thought many brilliant scholastic philosophers and theologians whose intellectual profundity was equal to the best, and better than most, of what followed. After all, the Scholastics labored on the fundamental questions all of their lives: the problem of being, knowledge and faith. In so far as they did so guided by commonly shared theological beliefs they have been slighted by the modern secularists. Yet they left both a rigorous method and a complex synthetic system.

The Medieval period is remembered because faith and reason met and did not find each other anathema. Such harmony was the fruit of the labors of the schoolmen and the natural philosophers within the church and despite the difficulties within the church in the fourteenth and fifteenth centuries, and the Reformation in the sixteenth, these centuries were still very much medieval in so far as the theological principle informed all activity. The possibilities for developments in science were only another expression of the values that Western civilization would take out of the Middle Ages, a civilization that would still be in every sense Christian, even when divided, and in every sense intellectual, even while Christian. The fact remains that no subsequent thinkers have pursued the intellectual life any more vigorously than the schoolmen, only in the modern age the goal of this activity shifted to positive knowledge and away from metaphysical problems. Yet the taking up of certain ideas and the abandoning of others does not indicate the superiority of modern intellectual life over the medieval. Nor should Scholasticism be discredited because it was not scientific. In the modern period we have accumulated an overabundance of knowledge without finding a corresponding way to put it in harmony with our existence. A new synthesis is possible, it is necessary, and it is inevitable. Perhaps rethinking Medieval thought will show us a way.

Early Modern Science

The fourteenth century witnessed a revival of interest in classical learning, a new focus on the things of this world, and the notion that though man serves a spiritual purpose as a member of the community of all men, he is also an individual who must maximize his talents for his own happiness and experience life's riches in his own way. Thus, Renaissance thinkers exhibited great interest in works which either hailed the idea of the individual or offered ample testimony to his genius. There were brilliant men in letters and the arts, and men of politics from whose pens the idea of nationhood and modern Europe would emerge. There were also leading men of trading and banking cities who presented the West its first genuine experiences with capitalism.

Men of science were less conspicuous and natural science fairly well remained in the hands of small numbers of individuals, while medicine continued as a discipline undertaken with great deference to the ancient wisdom. Neither medicine nor science in general advanced greatly on their own during the Renaissance, though they would later benefit from the intellectual freedom it announced, an extension of the idea that individual excellence most excellently accords with man's spiritual quest. The great men of the Renaissance were inspired men whose lives can hardly be appreciated if one restricts his observations to the technical side of their achievements, and these were not limited to the arts. Men such as Nicholas of Cusa and Leonardo da Vinci anticipated the evolution of modern science by advancing the idea that the scientist is also an artist, one who must pursue his intellectual craft with the same earnestness and self-confidence as other artists.

This view, held by Cusa and Leonardo, saw the scientist in possession of the key to nature in a special way, not merely receiving his impressions of nature passively, but recreating her as a reflection of their idea in the mind of God. As the intellect masters nature it moves toward God but under its own power, with its own categories and concepts. This is the Renaissance ideal of knowledge, concordant with both the mystical sense of God's work and the individual's power to know it and exalt it by his own efforts.

The Renaissance movement was a unifying force in southern Europe in so far as its artistic and individualistic spirit permeated the whole culture. In northern Europe, on the other hand, the Reformation crisis blunted its spirit and achievement while Reformation politics and theology overwhelmed cultural life. The Geneva of Calvin, the North Germany of Luther and the Scotland of Knox were places where life was harsh and its conduct strict. Any interest in the world in the sense that it was splendid or majestic was rare indeed. The resulting decline in cultural and intellectual life, then, placed the Protestant Reformation as something apart from the general spirit of Christian Europe, all of the latter's abuses notwithstanding. Science would need another century before medicine could lead a renewed interest in science and technology, but two great books did appear which foreshadowed the coming age of science. Copernicus and Vesalius were stimulated by their studies with Italian scientists and the congenial environment for making science; the authors were from the north but their books would have been impossible without the south.

The astronomical book, *De Revolutionibus,* was the capstone of Nicholas Copernicus's life work. Copernicus could not accept Ptolemy's cosmology placing the earth in the physical center of the system and the planets moving around it in a series of cycles and epicycles. Copernicus reasoned that Ptolemy's system was just too complex. The Creator, he thought, did not draw his plan from mathematical intricacies but from grand simplicity. Over the years of rethinking this cosmology Copernicus worked out a simpler mathematical arrangement which still satisfied the movements of the planets while introducing the heliocentric principle. Copernicus believed that the new astronomy reflected the intelligence of the Creator far better than the intricate system of the ancient star gazer. Yet as he lay near death, after his long labor, Copernicus was deeply anxious. For this devout man the publication of a book that profoundly altered the view of the relationship between sun and earth, man and cosmos, was momentous business. He wondered if God Himself would be displeased. Yet the more he pondered his own work the more he believed it reflected the grand design of the cosmos. Copernicus was a canon of the church, he had assisted Popes and bishops on scientific matters and dedicated this work, *De Revolutionibus,* to Paul III. He was sure that it would not subvert the faith but would enhance it by showing in the simplicity of planetary motion the harmony and economy of God's plan.

Copernicus had simplified the cosmic scheme by placing the earth in motion around the sun. He had worked without the telescope and his insights were of course not supportable by every day sense experience which had always suggested a sun in motion around a static earth. His works raised questions: the problem of parallax and the expected deflection of falling bodies from their straight line paths due to the new motions. Yet he advanced his theory, even without an answer to these objections, primarily because of his religious faith and his belief that it exalted the Creator of the heavens. On an early spring morning in 1543 a courier placed a copy of Copernicus's new book in the hands of the dying man. Copernicus uttered his last words "Lord, now I may depart in peace" and died an hour later.

Andreas Vesalius published *De Corpora Humana Fabrica* within months of Copernicus's death. *De Corpora* was the collection of Vesalius's public demonstrations in human anatomy which had made him the undisputed master of the art before he was thirty. His book was not only a brilliant intellectual achievement, it was an artistic one as well. Vesalius knew the artists in Titian's studio in Venice and had engaged one of them to illustrate the great work.

Long before the publication of *De Corpora,* Vesalius had set to work on his medical career. He had obtained his medical degree in Padua after leaving Venice and was invited to return as professor of anatomy. He had also studied at Louvain and at the greatest of the medieval universities, Paris, but he needed to breathe the intellectual air of Italy to bring his work into focus. Coming from a prominent line of medical people he also had the right connections. His great, great grandfather had translated the *Canons* of Avicenna, his great grandfather had been professor of medicine at Louvain, his father the court physician to Charles V. This distinguished lineage prepared him well for the greatness that waited.

De Corpora was the outstanding anatomical text up to its time and was one of the first truly scientific textbooks in any field. The brilliant illustrations by Kalcar added visual impact and beauty, assuring the book's lasting fame; the frontispiece powerfully depicted the new science: the splendor of the body, the skill of the anatomist, the intensity of the students. With *De Corpora* the doctor had become a scientist.

Vesalius, like Copernicus, studied the authorities and discovered many errors. Could it have been that Galen had not dissected the human body? Did the most famous doctor of antiquity make all of his observations from the dissection of apes? How could a man with the authority of 1400 years behind him be wrong? Vesalius corrected Galen because his was not human anatomy, just as Copernicus had to modify Ptolemy because of his geometrical complexity. Vesalius and Copernicus solved their dilemma in the same way. Their books would explicate the harmony in the cosmos and in the human form, respectively, and thereby reveal the magnificence of God's design.

Tyco Brahe took up the work of heliocentric cosmology after the death of Copernicus but it was Johannes Kepler who solved the mechanics of the Copernican system. Kepler was born in Wurtemburg in 1571. He studied philosophy and science at Tubingen and worked with Brahe at the end of the sixteenth century. In 1596 he published the *Mysterium Cosmographicum*, a mystical but yet not unreasonable view of the planetary arrangement. Kepler suggested that the distances among the five planets and the earth were proportional, arranged in a mathematical progression consistent with the configurations of the five regular solids. Kepler arrived at this because of his a priori view that the cosmos was mathematical and rational. Obviously, his arrangement was incorrect but it revealed Kepler's spiritual urges. Kepler also believed that his planetary arrangement had a relation to the musical scale and he wrote of the music spheres in another of his books, the *Harmonice Mundi*. These spiritual drifts were based on Kepler's belief in the divine economy in the heavens, even if this misrepresented it.

Kepler's lasting scientific contributions were defined in the *Astronomia Nova*. There Kepler noted that Mars moved in an elliptical orbit around the sun with a speed which increased as it approached the sun and decreased as it moved away. These observations were incorporated into a mathematical law of planetary motion; the square of the time of the revolutions of each of the planets was proportional to the cube of their mean distance from the sun. This mathematical principle of the solar system led to the refinements and advances of Galileo and the principle of gravity described by Isaac Newton.

Kepler was a religious man. He commented that God created the world in accordance with the principles of perfect numbers and it was for that reason that "the orbits are as they are." In a letter to his friend Johann Herwart he wrote, "we astronomers are priests of the most high God with respect to the book of nature,"[2] and that book of nature was mathematical. In defense of the Copernican teaching he wrote that the sun is the center "since it does not befit the first Mover to be diffused but to proceed from one certain principle; by the highest right we return to the sun who's essence is pure light, who alone appears suited to become the home of God himself."[3] This is mystical science and the notion of "the essence of pure light" good Platonic metaphysics. Thus Kepler had no difficulty in writing in his *Harmonice Mundi* that astrology has direct effects on the world and on human events as when eclipses, constellations, and comets announce great events in the political realm or the position of the planets at one's birth affected the composition of humours. He believed that comets came directly from God and were the Divine intervention in the affairs of men, noting they had preceeded the births of Alexander, Mithradates and Mohammed. Finally, Kepler believed that underlying all things was a soul of the whole universe, a divine principle that informed, governed and sustained the cosmic arrangement, a view held by Pythagoras and Plato and later by Leibniz, Hegel, and Chardin.

Galileo Galilei was less of a mystic than Kepler but no less religious, though he has gone down in history as the St. George of science fighting the dragon of Curial reaction. Like Kepler, he was influenced by the geometrical atomism in Plato's *Timeaus* and Plato's mathematical metaphysics. Galileo believed that bodies had an infinite number of atoms and that all things in nature were made up of atoms in mathematical proportions. His metaphysics and his physics were based on the belief that God made the world mathematically and measurable in time and space. Galileo, of course, was nurtured in Christian belief and in no way sought to overturn it. He rather argued, as he did in his letters to the Grand Dutchess Christine, the wife of his benefactor Cosimo DeMedici, that science approached openly and with the desire for the truth would confirm revelation:

> I think that in discussions of physical problems we ought to begin not from scripture but from sense experience and necessary demonstrations. For the Holy Bible and the phenomena of nature proceed alike from the divine word. The former as the dictate of the spirit and the latter as the observant executrix of God's commands. Nor is God any less excellently revealed in nature's action than in the sacred statements of the Bible.[4]

Galileo also quoted Tertullian, "We conclude that God is known first through nature and then again, more particularly, by doctrine; by nature in his works, and by doctrine in his revealed word."[5] The problem as Galileo saw it was that revelation must also be understood without the confusions that run whilly nilly contrary to reason when reason is served in revelation. For Galileo, then, the issue wasn't revelation, but interpretation. Seeing as he lived during the Reformation such concern was reasonable especially as both religion and science were giving men a basis for reinterpreting the more obscure passages of the Holy book.

Galileo is best remembered atop the tower at Pisa dropping his weights to the ground and measuring their time of impact or gazing at the swinging lantern in the cathedral at Pisa, noting that it took the same time for each oscillation even as the distance through each oscillation decreased as the pendulum slowed. Such keenness of insight and observation, time and again marks Galileo as one of the giants of the scientific method. It also makes him an interesting subject for any student of the intellectual processes of the scientist. Clearly Galileo, like Newton and Kepler, was not a man who could be simply labelled; no strict inductionist or deductionist was he, but possessed of great intellectual vision that lead to those inspirations which cap years of patient toil.

In 1604 Galileo, then in Padua, discovered a new star, confirming Tyco's notion that there were events in the cosmos beyond the solar system that were changing and could only be explained by a dynamic universe. This discovery refuted Aristotle's static universe just as Galileo's observations on the acceleration of falling bodies had refuted his mechanics. On the early morning of January 7, 1610 Galileo observed what he at first thought to be four new planets which he called the Medicean Planets after Cosimo. In the next several days Galileo realized that they revolved around Jupiter, an important observation further confirming the Copernican view. Galileo announced these findings as well as his work on sunspots and the topography of the moon in his book the *Nuncius Siderius*, "the Starry messenger."

Galileo visited Rome in 1615 and was counseled as to the philosophical cracks in his theories. He was not, however, forbidden to continue his teaching if it should be qualified as theory. In 1629 he published the *Dialogues on the Two Chief Systems* which added more support to Copernicus while adding a theory which largely anticipated Newton's first law, the law of inertia. In 1632 he was recalled to Rome and censored for his Copernicanism although many historians of the event attribute his problems to his remonstrances in *The Dialogue* presented through the voice of the enlightened Copernican, Salviati, against Simplicio, the reactionary Aristotelian, Pope Urban VII. It was, perhaps, this ill considered incivility that found Galileo in the Office of the Inquisition. This time his books were banned and he was placed in confinement. Later he returned to his country estate and lived out the remainder of his life performing many experiments, finally publishing his *Nova Scientia* in Leyden in 1638. In this work Galileo presented the revolutionary idea of accelerated velocity which explained many of his experiments with falling bodies and bodies on inclined planes.

The culmination of this work on planetary mechanics came with Isaac Newton's *Principia Mathematica* in 1687, and the law of universal gravity. Newton had already worked for many years on the foundations laid by Copernicus, Kepler and Galileo and within the same world view. Newton, too, understanding creation as a rational exercise knowable through mathematical and geometrical measurements, its mechanics reducible to simple laws.

Newton was born in 1643 and was educated at Trinity College, Cambridge. Early on he had an interest in physical theories and worked with spectrum analysis, color formation and astronomy. In his early twenties he had conceived the idea of universal gravity although many years of observation and experiment would pass before he could publish it in its mathematical form. He did write sometime in 1665 that gravity presented itself to him based on Kepler's observations on planetary motion: "I deduced from Kepler's rules of the periodical times of the planets that the force which keeps the planets in their orbs must be reciprocally as the squares of their distance from the center."[5] Thus the planetary motions that Kepler and Copernicus had observed but could not explain based on a physical law was now understood to be a consequence of gravity. Gravity would become the universal law for motions of bodies in the cosmos.

Newton was deeply indebted to those who had worked before him. Borelli had studied centrifugal force while the Dutch physicist, Christian Huygens, came close to a theory of gravity when discussing the force that kept planets from flying away from the sun. Huygens observed the acceleration of a body in motion in a circle and had developed a mathematical formula for acceleration towards the center for revolving bodies which Edmund Halley, of the comet, had also anticipated. William Gilbert, the physician who had announced the principle of the magnet in 1600, pondered the question as to the nature of the force accounting for magnetism. Gilbert's immediate answer was that it was all some occult force, the relationships between magnetic bodies was a relationship mysteriously aligned to a soul principle, not unlike the great soul of the universe that Kepler had announced in his *Harmonice Mundi.*

Newton put it all together. By the time of the *Principia* he had formulated the three laws of motion: the law of inertia which had been anticipated by Galileo, the law of gravity, and the law of equal and opposite reaction. These laws became the basis for the mechanical universe of experimental science and physics for the next 250 years. At the same time Newton stated the theological beliefs implied in his science. He wrote theological treatises arguing that natural law is a manifestation of God's law. Above all, he saw in the workings of the physical universe the very principle of reason. He would ask, as he did in his *Optics:*

> To what end are comets and whence is it that planets move all one and the same in orbs concentric, and what hinders the fixed stars from falling upon one another, how came the bodies of animals to be contrived with so much art and for what ends were their several parts. Was the eye contrived without skill in optics or the ear without knowledge of sounds/ And all these things being rightly dispatched does it not appear from phenomena that there is a being incorporeal, living, intelligent, omnipresent, who in infinite

space sees the things intimately and thoroughly perceives them
and comprehends them only by their immediate presence to
Himself?[6]

The thrust of natural philosophy was directed towards ascertaining these
natural laws. It was not merely fortuitous, then, that late in the sixteenth
century, before Newton and Galileo, the principle of natural law was once
again articulated by Richard Hooker. Hooker's work *The Laws of Ecclesiastical
Polity* was published in 1595, almost fifty years before Newton's birth. It
began with an important statement regarding natural law, though Hooker
largely confined its application to his defense of the Anglican church. Hooker
stated that natural law governs the cosmos, natural phenomena and human
behavior, a reflection of a view already maturing in the latter sixteenth century as a legacy of Aristotle and the Scholastics, and a presentiment of the
natural philosophy and the political thought of the seventeenth and
eighteenth centuries. Hooker wrote:

> All things that are have some operation not violent or casual.
> Neither doth any thing ever begin to exercise the same without
> some fore conceived end for which it worketh...that which doth
> appoint the form and measure of working, the same we term a law.
> *Hooker goes on:* neither have they other wise spoken of that cause
> than as an agent which knowing what and why it worketh obser-
> veth in working a most exact order or law.[7]

Hooker notes that his is what Homer mentioned, this was acknowledged by
Hermes Trismegistus, Anaxagoras and Plato

> terming the maker of the world an intelligent worker. Finally, all
> confessed therefore in the working of the first cause, that counsel is
> used, reason followed, a way observed which is a constant order
> and law that is kept whereof itself must needs be author unto
> itself.[8]

Hooker pointed out that the first principles of reason are self-evident. If
this were not so then we remove all possibilities for knowing anything, as
Aristotle noted. Hooker's was a sixteenth century answer to the twentieth
century positivists who reduce knowledge to knowledge based solely on
experience and the verification principle.

> And herein Theophrastus is true. They that seek a reason of all
> things do what only overthrows reason. In every kind of knowl-
> edge some such grounds there are as that being proposed the mind
> doth presently embrace them as free from all possibilities of error
> clear and manifest without proof.[9]

Hooker gained more renown as a philosophical father to such political thinkers as John Locke and Edmund Burke than as a natural scientist, but his "natural law" views saw much wider application, implicit even in the science of the seventeenth century.

If developments in astronomy heralded in *De Revolutionibus* in 1543 and climaxed by Newton's *Principia* in 1687 are major events in the rise of modern science, they still do not eclipse the equally important advances in medicine, anatomy and physiology that were being made in Italy before Copernicus. In fact, much of the credit for methodology and attention to careful experiment that marks good science was the result of those efforts in medicine and biology. Indeed, the great theorems of astronomy were a purely intellectual piece whereas the knowledge gained from the dissection table and the physiology room was directly observable. Experimental and laboratory work, then, grew as the interests of those practicing dissection and studying the mechanics of the body worked to correct Galen and others. Even Galileo learned his methods as a medical student, under Cesalpinus, and by the time of publication of Vesalius' *Fabric of the Human Body* anatomy had helped establish the new methods in science.

Galen had been a good observer in his own right and had experimented, but he had not opened the human body. Human anatomy really begins in the fifteenth century in Italy. This is the anatomy of Taddeo Mondino, who published the first true anatomical text in Bologna, and Anthony Bienvieni at Florence who anticipated Morgagni with his interest in pathological anatomy. Bienvieni noted that in observing disease we must search out the seat of it, making that principle the basis of his anatomical dissection. Leonardo daVinci was also a distinguished anatomist proposing a theory of the circulation and illustrating in the greatest detail the structure of muscles and bones. He was one of the first to begin the departure from the Galenical tradition and he was the first to make waxen casts of organs.

Post-Vesalian anatomy was especially lively in Padua, Bologna and the Papal Medical School and through Colombo, Eustachi, Fallopius, and Fabricius of Aquapendente (the anatomist at Padua who taught William Harvey, which led to Harvey's classic *De Motu Cordis,* describing the circulation of the blood and the motion of the heart). Actually, Cesalpino of Pisa, a papal physician, taught the circulation of the blood before Harvey published his work, maintaining that the heart was the seat of the vital principle, the anima, and the great organ of sanquification. We should not fail to mention that Michael Servetus had arrived at a theory of the circulation before Cesalpino and Harvey. Servetus had a knowledge of the pulmonary circulation in the middle of the sixteenth century, gained after studying at Paris and working with DuBois and Fernel. Servetus' promising career met an untimely end on the block, however. He was executed for a theological heresy by John Calvin at Geneva in 1553.

The interest in anatomy and physiology in Italy during the sixteenth-eighteenth centuries was in good measure due to the enlightened reception given anatomical science by the Popes. The Popes, after all, shared the views of the natural philosophers, astronomers and physicians about science and Divine reason and many of the best anatomists and physicians of this period were papal physicians. During this time dissection was usually conducted as a public event with ceremony and ritual on Feast days or holidays with civic and church leaders in attendance. A lecturer would read from the texts of the ancient masters while a "prosector" performed the dissection and a "demonstrator" exhibited the specific parts to the audience. All of this, of course, refutes the view that a decree of Pope Boniface VIII in the beginning of the fourteenth century interdicted human anatomy. Boniface wished only to forbid the mangling of the body and the careless treatment of the remains. The decree did not forbid dissection conducted under the guidelines set forth by Boniface. In fact, soon after, Mondino established the Medical School at Bologna as the leading center for anatomical studies and Guy de Chauliac, the greatest surgeon of the day, came there to study.

The papal interest in medicine had been in evidence well before the fourteenth century. In the eleventh century Pope Victor III wrote a treatise on medicine while he was a member of the Order of St. Benedict. Peter the Spaniard, later Pope John XXI, was a trained physician who taught physiology at the University of Siena and wrote a textbook on diet and surgery. He was also considered an authority on diseases of the eye. Innocent III established the city hospitals and brought Guy of Montpeilier, a leading physician of his time, to Rome to help establish the hospital San Spirito. And the pope who supposedly outlawed dissection was operated on by one of the great physicians of his century, Arnold of Villanova, the Pope's lithotomist. Clearly, a pope who submitted to the knife was not likely to use a surgeon who didn't know where to place it!

The spirit of scientific investigation, therefore, was alive and well in Italy and the receptivity of the Church to the advancement of learning was a major factor. A term of study in Italy was obligatory for the scientists from other countries who wished to learn new techniques and advance their scholarship and among them was the esteemed William Harvey.

Harvey delivered the Lumleian lectures before the College of Physicians, London, in April of 1616. Here, for the first time, he publically presented his theory of the circulation. The evidence he brought on its behalf was impressive indeed, including the records of his dissections of the valves of the veins which directed flow of blood to the heart, the relation of the contraction of the heart to the propagation of the pulse and the relation between lung function and blood flow. Harvey's belief in the order of nature and the human body overcame the doubts other anatomists had regarding the knowledge of the heart. They believed its secrets would forever be known only to God. Harvey believed otherwise: nature would reveal her laws if one pursued nature with a lover's earnestness. The anatomist must go right to nature and find there God's design:

> I profess to learn and teach not from books but from dissection, not from the tenets of philosophers but from the fabric of nature.[10]

The blood, then, was only as it could be, the most harmonious and ordered of all movements in nature and cosmos, and Harvey found it such because he believed it to be so. He was no mere technician, he had a mystical feel for his work, as Abraham Cowley implied in his poem, "Upon Dr. Harvey":

> The heart of man, what art can ere reveal
> a wall impervious between divides the very parts within,
> and does the heart of man even from itself conceal.
> She spoke but ere she was aware,
> Harvey was with her there.[11]

The Harveian tradition continued with Thomas Willis who described the circulation of the brain working with Christopher Wren who made the copper plates for Willis' books, Richard Lower, the first Englishman to perform a blood transfusion, and that superb practitioner of the scientific method, Robert Boyle.

Boyle was a member of an illustrious group of experimentors and natural philosophers, the "invisibles," who met regularly at Gresham College in London to discuss their scientific works. The group finally became an official body, the Royal Society, in 1662, receiving its charter from Charles II. Boyle, himself, had become interested in anatomy and physiology as a student of Sir William Petty, the physician to Cromwell's Army in Ireland, and then as a student of Petty's cousin, Nathaniel Highmore. Boyle wrote extensively on natural philosophy, medicine and theology and performed many experiments, among the best entered in the proceedings of the Royal Society in their publication, *The Philosophical Transactions*. In his least known but important work, *The Christian Virtuoso,* Boyle announced that "by being addicted to experimental philosophy a man is rather assisted than indisposed to be a good Christian."[12] He felt strongly that the study of nature was the study of the Divine plan. The "Virtuoso" was its student, one accomplished in the scientific methods and moved by his religious belief. Boyle is one of the founders of modern chemistry and physiology along with Jean Baptiste VonHelmont who shared Boyle's views on the beauty and rationality of nature and the importance of investigations in natural philosophy.

The successes in anatomy and physiology in the seventeenth and eighteenth centuries captured the imagination of thinkers in all fields and the medical model, the harmony and order of the human body, was held out as a model for the political and social arrangement as well. Indeed, some physicians distinguished themselves in these fields using their medical experience to frame their philosophical and political insights. William Petty, John Locke and Francois Quesnay were among the most famous of these "natural law" theorists.

Petty began his career as the chief physician for the armies of Parliament. He was appointed surveyor general of Ireland and his work there led him to economics, and he was one of the first to present the labor theory of value and the concept of differential rent, important principles of classical economics in England. One modern student of economics noted that the three great forces of scientific methodology, natural law theory and economic analysis, were uniquely joined in Petty. Petty was the English equivalent of the physiocrat, strongly arguing that the economical base of a nation was in its land and agricultural development, and his Political Arithmetic was one of the first treatises to measure the relative wealth of the nations of Europe and England, and the first to apply statistical methods. His treatise on taxes was the first to suggest a proportional taxation of properties and incomes. As befits a physician, he gave a physiological summation of the role of government in the economical activity of the state

> that as wiser physicians tamper not excessively with their patients
> rather observing and complying with the motions of nature than
> contradicting it with vehement administrations of their own, so in
> politics and economics the same must be used.[13]

John Locke followed Petty's empirical tradition. Locke was also a physician, an Oxford scientist, friend of the Royal Society and favorite of the Earl of Shaftsbury. Throughout most of his life Locke maintained a correspondence with Sydenham in which they discussed medicine, politics and religion and as a result of an early correspondence Locke had correctly judged that his benefactor, Shaftsbury, was suffering from an amebic liver abscess. Locke assisted in the management of the case, the first reported drainage of such an abscess, and a grateful Earl made him his advisor on economics and politics. As a result Locke became world famous as the classical "natural right" theorist and political defender of property and person.

Francois Quesnay, a French surgeon and medical writer, was court physician to Madame Pompadour and Louis XV. He wrote a political classic,

Tableau Economique, outlining the principle programs of the French economy establishing him as one of the founders of the physiocratic movement, representing many of the distinguished political and economical figures of eighteenth century France including the Marquis de Mirabeau, Mercier de la Riviere, DuPont DeNemours, of the famous DuPonts, and Anne Marie de Turgot. As "physiocrats" they took the perfectly executing model of the human body with its physiological laws as the model for the ideal economic and political community. This was not unreasonable as astronomers, physicists and physicians were describing both the cosmos and the body according to the ordered natural law. At the same time each advance in human anatomy and physiology affirmed anew the ordered body. Naturally enough, men projected the political arrangement as a "body politic" with its inherent rationality (if only it were true).

While some medical men made their names in economics and politics, others worked in conjunction with scientists and statesmen to promote new scientific societies such as the Berlin Academy, the Institutes in Rome and Florence and the Royal Society in London, already mentioned. The Royal Society was the first of these to publish a house organ, *The Philosophical Transactions,* which treated questions in natural philosophy and advances in medicine and biology. The entries were diverse, some scholarly and original, some entertaining and some showing the downright gullibility of the men of early modern science. The "transactions" included entries on new anatomical discoveries and findings related to post mortem examinations. One paper described the autopsy exam of Malphigi, the anatomist who discovered the capillary system, thus completing Harvey's theory of the circulation. The autopsy, conducted by Lancisi, notes that Malphigi forbade his friends to open his body until thirty hours after his death for, "he knew well enough that some who seemed dead have revived some hours after." Perhaps Malphigi had recalled such experiences in his own dissecting and Vesalius is remembered to have ceased his anatomical dissections after he opened the cadaver of a prisoner and found the heart still beating. He made a hasty penitent's retreat to the Holy Land thinking he had anatomized a living subject and died from an infectious disease on his journey home.

The experiments recorded in *The Transactions* were vivid and colorful, especially those on breathing and circulation by Lower, Hooke and Boyle. Boyle described experiments in which he kept his dogs breathing with the assistance of a bellows, describing the convulsive fits that would ensue when the bellows were deflated. Hooke mentions a similar experiment:

> I formerly tried keeping a dog alive after his thorax was all displayed but diverse persons seeming to doubt of the certainty of the experiment, I caused it to be repeated at the meeting of the Society

with the same success, the dog being kept alive by the reciprocal blowing up of his lungs with bellows and then suffered to subside for the space of an hour or more after his thorax had been so displayed. The dog having been thus kep 'live in which time the trial was often repeated and suffering the dog to fall into convulsive -motions by ceasing to blow the bellows and then of a sudden reviving him again by renewing the blast and consequently the motion of the lungs. I conclude that as the bare motion of the lungs without fresh air contributes nothing to the life of the animal it was not the subsiding or motionlessness that was the immediate cause of death or the stopping of the circulation of the blood through the lungs but the wont of sufficient supply of fresh air.[14]

In an experiment which would have put to rest Malphigi's anxieties, a Mr. Templer describes how he "cut out the heart of two urchins and found the systole and diastole to continue a full two hours while the hearts lay upon a glazed earthen white plate in a cold window."[15] Templer asks "When shall we say any animal or insect is dead if it hath motion?"[16]

Pepys, the chronicler, described many Royal Society experiments including Lower's transfusion experiments. Pepys noted that the first transfusion of blood from one dog into another had been made for the society by Thomas Cox and a Mr. King, repeating an experiment that had been coached by Robert Boyle and conducted by Dr. Lower. In *The Transactions* Lower described the procedure:

I first take up the carotid artery of the dog and separate it from the nerves and lay it bare, then make a long ligature in the upper part of the artery and about an inch below towards the heart make another ligature of a running knot. Having made these two knots draw two threads under the artery and put a quill in and tie the artery upon the quill. After this make bare jugular vein in the other dog and at each end make a ligature with a running knot and in the space betwixt the two running knots draw the vein under two threads as in the other. Then make an incision in the vein and put into it two quills one into the descendant part of the vein to receive the blood from the other dog and carry it to the heart and the other quill put into the other part of the vein out of which the second dogs own blood must run into dishes. All things being thus prepared fasten the dogs on their sides towards one another so that the quills may go into each other. After that unstop the quill that goes down into the first dog's vein and the other quill coming out of the other dogs artery and by the help of two of the other quills put into each other according as there shall be occasion insert them into one another then slit the running knots and immediately the blood runs the quills as through an artery very impetuously.[15]

Christopher Wren had described infusions of drugs and poisons before Lower's experiments. The French, however, credited their Jean Denis for transfusing blood between animals a year before Lower's experiment. The transfusion experiments raised the old questions about the anima, the life force or vital principle. Boyle had asked whether "by transfusion of blood the disposition of individuals of the same kind may not be much altered." He questioned whether a fierce dog by being transfused with the blood of a cowardly dog may not become more tame, whether a transfused dog will recognize his master, or characteristics peculiar to a breed would be abolished or impaired. Boyle even wondered if rejuvenation would occur if an old dog was given the blood of a vigorous one. Out of all of this work, came new theories about the blood and the heart as the source of life and emotions. There was furious speculation about the humours, behavior and temperament, and the relationship between emotions, disease and the circulation of the vital principle. But none of these experimenters freed themselves of the notion of spiritual essences as part of the human physiology. Harvey himself had believed in an ethereal essence that was somehow carried with the vital principle and was incorporated into the heat of the body, either as spontaneous heat or heat brought by the spirit itself, accounting for emotions, an idea which prevailed among society members including Boyle, Hooke, Lower and Wren.

The first animal transfusions were followed up by the first human transfusions. Lower conducted the experiment in 1667 and it was described in a letter to Robert Boyle by another observer. He noted that Dr. Lower and Dr. King had given the blood of a young sheep to the quantity of about eight or nine ounces into the great vein of the arm of a man. The letter goes on:

> The patient found himself better than before...and more composed, he being looked upon before as a very freakish man who had studied at Cambridge and is said to be a bachelor of Divinity, an indigent, receiving a guinea for undergoing the experiment, which reward maketh him willing to have it repeated upon him.[16]

The Transactions record other curious transfusion experiments. There was a paper "The transfusion of the blood of a mangee into a found dog" by Mr. Theodore Cox who writes

> that the effect of this experiment was no alteration at all to be observed in the found dog but for the mangee dog, he was in about ten days or a fortnights space perfectly cured.[17]

There is the transfusion of the blood of a young into an old dog by Mr. Gayant who notes:

> The blood of a young dog having been given into the veins of an old, which two hours after did leap and frisk whereas he was almost blind with age and could hardly stir before.[18]

And a description of the transfusion of the blood of calves into dogs by Jean Denis:

> Since the ninth of March 1666-1667 we have transfused the blood of three calves into three dogs after which the dogs did eat as well as before and one of the three dogs from which so much blood had been drawn the day before that he could hardly stir anymore, having been supplied the next morning with the blood of a calf recovered instantly his strength and showed a surprising vigor.[19]

The transfusion of the blood of a lamb into a spaniel led to the most fanciful claim. The spaniel had been

> noted to be of middle size, thirteen years old and altogether deaf for above three years. He walked very little and was so feeble that he was unable to lift his feet. After the transfusion, in two days he was running up and down the streets with other dogs without trailing his feet as he did before, his stomach also returned to him and he began to eat more greedily than before, but that which is more surprising is that from that time he gave signs that he began to hear, returning sometimes at the voice of his master.[20]

No wonder the blood was the "vita anima!"

Obviously, such descriptions, imaginative though they were, hardly deterred people now interested in the new sciences. Thus it is no surprise that the medical scene was generously populated with quacks, charlatans and glib purveyors, and much healing remained in the hands of "common artificers."

Valentine Greatrakes, an Irish volunteer in Cromwell's army, was one of the most famous of these healers, claiming the function of the "Royal touch," part of healing since the days of Edward the Confessor when monarchs laid hands on thousands of their subjects to remove the curse of tuberculosis. *The Transactions* described the work of the "Stroake," Greatrakes:

> When he stroake for pain he useth his dry hand, if ulcers or running sores, spittle. For the evil he ordered it poulticed with boiled turnips, then lanced it and squeezed out the cores and corruption.[21]

Greatrakes may have been one of the more legitimate healers—at least he drained wounds. Most offered only empty words and worthless remedies, "practitioners who, with a trunk full of nostrums, bid disease to vanish and death retire from the scenes of their triumphs." Both rich and poor, royalty and common folk were called to cures. The Quacks were impressive enough to entice most anyone by accumulating the usual requisites, a decent black suit or a plush though slightly worn jacket and a carriage and a footman if one were successful. The Quack was well advised to walk with gravity as in "deep contemplation upon arbitrament between life and death." He should also "keep nearby a skeleton to proclaim a skill in anatomy" and he should "fail not to oblige ale houses to recommend inquirers and ask nurses and midwives to applaud his skills at gossipings."[22] Even Queen Anne was taken in. Cursed with poor eyesight, she offered position and money to any who promised relief. One William Asade, previously a tailor, rose to knighthood by her hand and put out a book of "All Diseases incident to the eye" even though he could not read. Sir William, joined by Roger Grant, a cobbler and Anabaptist preacher, were two of the Queen's "sworn oculists," publishing detailed accounts of their "cures" and soliciting written testimony from the healed, routine practice among quacks.[23]

One of the preeminent charlatans of the day was Thomas Saffold. Formerly a weaver, he graduated to cures and prognostications and paid shills and bill distributors to work the crowds along Cheapside and the Strand, praising his healing and speaking of his cures in colorful verse. Nor did the certified doctors of the time abjure such methods. Sir Edward Hannes, M.D., a contemporary of Radcliffe and King, was in the custom of sending footmen on before him to poke their heads into every coach anxiously inquiring as to the whereabouts of the good doctor who was urgently needed. Like the quacks, the physicians dressed to success, a proper wig, fine cloth, polished canes, preferably with gold heads, and a coach and a fine team if the fees were good. Certainly quacks and regualr physicians were accused of loving nothing but their fees and both could be terribly indelicate about collecting.

John Radcliffe, M.D., a notoriously stingy man, once treated a patient for free for twelve months as promised, but when the year lapsed and patient offered the entire fee in gold coin, Radcliffe weakened and turned his palm saying, "Singly, Sir, I could have refused, but all together, they are irresistible.[24] Sir Richard Jebb, once expecting five guineas as a fee, seeing only three were paid, dropped the coins and as he slowly picked them up looked about for two more telling his patient that he was sure he would not have quibbled the additional two—the hint was taken. Another doctor of the time was reported to have come upon the bedside of a dead patient, whereupon he found the man's hand closed around a gold coin. This physician calmly announced "Ah, that was for me, clearly,"[25] as he put the piece in his pocket. Even then death did not relieve you of your financial obligation!

The eighteenth century was equally graced with dubious healers and methods. Perhaps the greatest stir was created by Franz Anton Mesmer,

M.D., by way of Vienna, who arrived in Paris in the latter part of the century working hypnotic therapies. His "Aimal Magnetism" was especially popular since Gilbert's theory of the magnet had described force acting at a distance. Mesmer was a force himself and his performances in Paris were so popular that the French Government offered him the Cross of the Order of St. Michael for his secret. His following didn't last, however, and he was finally pronounced a fraud by a group that included Benjamin Franklin, who noted that "Most of the women who presented themselves to be magnetized came out of idleness or amusement...and the action of the imagination produced a certain disorder throughout the machine."[26]

Robert Falbor hawked a secret remedy, an extract of Peruvian bark, with such grand claims that he was made court physician to Charles II. Later he sold his formula to Louis XIV for an annuity and a title. A devious widow, Joanna Stephens, successfully hawked her cure for bladder stones, a concoction which included roasted egg shells and garden snails. The Prime Minister, Walpole, swore by the widow's remedy and took it "by the pound." Count Cagliostro, erstwhile thief and forger, arrived in London to evade the Italian authorities and won wide acclaim for his panacea and youth potion. James Graham, M.D., observed Benjamin Franklin's experiments with electricity when he visited the United States. The good doctor saw some possibilities there, and upon his return to London he opened Graham's "Temple for Health" in which wired chairs and soft music were used, while the doorways were framed by the discarded crutches of the cured. Graham's most innovative move was to promote his "celestial bed" to which barren couples were urged to repair. Graham was not to be outdone, however, and soon one Elisha Perkins of New Haven established himself as the king of appliance healing with his metallic tractors, two metallic rods drawn over the skin of the sick to lift diseases out of the body. The metallic rods were supposed to provide an electric impulse but cost considerations did allow for the introduction of wooden rods in the Perkin's clinic in London.

We may smile at these foibles, but the unfailing need for cures and the unflinching beliefs in all promises of the same have been an intimate part of the medical story of all ages, including our own. Lord Bacon, himself not wholly removed from chicanery, said it best:

> The physician, and the politician, is judged most by the event, for who can tell if a patient die or recover, or a state be preserved or received, whether it be art or accident? And therefore many times the impostor is prized and the man of virtue taxed.[27]

Quacks, frauds and clumsy physicians allowed, there still could be no turning back from the advance of science and medicine during this period and though there is little question that the scientists of the time kept their theology, the new knowledge was specifically removed from faith and revelation and as theological principles began to recede in the face of rational ones, knowledge was increasingly evaluated on its own merit and the desire for confirmatory research and scientific scrutiny only grew stronger. Theology was not yet under siege but it would less and less be sought as an explanation. Once science provided demonstrated knowledge mens' affections logically would pass over the indemonstrable.

The results of this progress in the seventeenth century in England led to a movement specifically disengaging itself from the indemonstrable. Deism, of course, was not in any sense a denial of God, but it clearly denied that we could prove Him. The emphasis on reason and experience so evident in Locke and Hobbes and the cornerstone of Hume's philosophy in the eighteenth century indicated the directions of philosophical thought in an age busy making science. The English Deists, beginning with Lord Herbert and followed by Tindal, Bolingbruke and Toland, emphasized a God of nature. From now on it would be ridiculous to talk of miracles, spirits, or invisible forces of the theological kind. God is in nature, but nature works on her own, through fixed laws, originally given by the Author of all but then removed from Him.

The Deists still professed a belief in the Almighty but their business was with nature, her first principles, her laws, her control through reason. Yet Hume, the crown prince of the English enlightenment, was less certain of all this talk of knowledge through reason and questioned the assumption that the fruits of reason are certain and irrefutable. Hume's scepticism was incongenial to science but it was also a natural outgrowth of the drift toward an eighteenth century positivism. All of this influenced the Enlightenment on the continent where the encyclopedists appealed to deistic thinking, Hume's scepticism and Newton's Physics in their own emphasis on reason and new knowledge. The "Philosophes" were desirous of applying reason and science to psychology and social theory, marking them as an important force in separating all intellectual pursuits from any formal theological considerations. But all of this was a gradual process and the work of individuals more than a specific movement. The complete separation of science from religion lay a century ahead with wider acceptance of science and the unarguable success of the new knowledge in defining and controlling biological and physical events.

Eighteenth - Nineteenth Century

Renaissance Italy and Reformation Europe produced some great names in science but more widespread interest in the methods and possibilities for science came after the work of Descartes, Bacon and Newton, while psychology and epistemology developed with the English Empiricists Locke and Hume. Frances Bacon made an important contribution with his emphasis on the inductive method. Bacon believed that nature could be understood (and mastered) by the accumulation of facts gained through careful research. The English devotion to empiricism ran strong in Bacon and lent great impetus to the study of nature separate from spirit or vitalism. Perhaps more importantly, Bacon preached the idea that science is power, the key to the control of nature and the advancement of society, an idea which would be given a more sinister cast in the twentieth century by another Englishman, Houston Chamberlain.

Across the channel from the England of Bacon, Rene Descartes enunciated another important working principle for science. His distinction between mind (spirit) and matter formed the basis for a great deal of subsequent scientific thinking. Descartes' method and philosophy emphasized that matter was a separate reality from the activity of the mind though ultimately connected to it by God's design. Descartes said that the mind (soul) works through the principles of motion and is thus dependent on matter. He based his physiology on the confluence of motions in the nervous system and the action of diverse animal spirits which are linked by their common center of activity in the soul (the pineal gland). Descartes, of course, never doubted that the origin of spirit (and matter) lay in the realm of God, nonetheless his notion of matter-extension and his intellectual methods were later interpreted to promote the propositions that matter and spirit were irreconcilable principles. If the scientific view which followed could be properly called Cartesian (it can't) it is the result of that proposition yet Descartes was no materialist and his methodologic doubt was not meant to vanquish spirit. His method was essentially deductionist and intuitive, a comprehensive system based on the "cogito" principle. "I think" and I know that I do, therefore my intellectual contemplation of nature is not self deceiving. Likewise, nature can be defined in a geometrical structure, in harmony with God's design, and this can lead to the idea of God's existence through the existence of the self-evident "cogito."

The beginning of the eighteenth century brought still greater emphasis on reason while allowing that God had something to do with the world. By the end of the century, however, reason claimed the highest value for itself. Rationalism, the condition of accepting knowledge verified through the resources of intellect and the mind's criteria was a first principle. It quickly gained both as a philosophy and as a method even though arguments raged as to whether it was the criteria, the phenomena, or things in themselves which were the source of knowledge. Likewise, new knowledge was also sought by accummulating facts from observation and the application of methods without invoking grand deductive systems. This is not to say that the "philosophes," the writers in the French Enlightenment of mid century, were strict empiricists or rationalists but they were certainly agreed that both would bring a new order. This tended to obscure the differences between the rationalists and the empiricists and it did help set reason free. First, however, reason had to loosen its connection from loftier thought. God, freedom and immortality were imponderables so reason had to efface them. Yet the philosophes were not dogmatic atheists either, excepting perhaps D'Holbach and LaMettrie, anymore than they were strict materialists. Their interest was the progress of the race through reason, in the social and political world and in science, a science of experience built on observation which would be descriptive rather than aprioristic. This is one of the main reasons why the French exhibited such a keen interest in the English, especially Bacon, Newton and Locke while rejecting any grand theories of nature as those of Leibniz, Spinoza and Descartes with their implied metaphysics.

The Encyclopedists, the authors of the bible of reason in mid-century, believed that Newton and Locke, far more than Descartes, had presented the appropriate approach to science (the methods of Bacon) because neither Locke nor Newton would hazard metaphysical speculations. Locke, for instance, was careful in his psychology to remove innate ideas and aprioristic principles and to argue that knowledge is developed through sensation (an act of the senses) and perception (intellectual quantification of the sense data).

Here was good empirical thinking that lent itself to careful science, in the encyclopedists' view. Newton, of course, was the finest exemplar of this empirical excellence but the encyclopedists failed to recognize that Newton's method was only comprehensible by use of a mathematics which itself was removed from any array of inductive experiences. Newton, like Galileo who Goethe said was that "genius for whom one case stands for a thousand," made an intellectual leap far beyond the mere quantification of empirical data.

Nonetheless, facts were the important commodity in the new science; theories would now begin to rise or fall on the solid witness of experimental validity and empirical consistency, the kinds of approaches which highlight modern science. Ernst Cassirer noted the important change that took place during the Enlightenment:

> The certainty of facts (had been) subordinated to that of the principles and dependent on the latter. The new physical theory which owes its existence to Newton and Locke, reverses this, the principle is derivative, the fact, as such, is original.[1]

Actually, Newton and Locke, and hardly alone, still kept the metaphysical order of things. What came after Newton and Locke, and not necessarily because of them, was the eventual dissolution of the theological principle. Both would have found that unacceptable as they still held that God was the unstated explanation for physical law and political principle respectively. Yet their efforts in physics and psychology, directed to descriptive knowledge and the facts of the experience separate from metaphysical causes or first principles did articulate the ideal scientific inquiry, an ideal taken further as it passed through the hands of the Dutch, the French and then the German natural philosophers and scientists. Through these passages theological explanations gradually receded as explanations for the events in nature. Few of the Enlightenment figures themselves denied belief but they made it possible for reason to eliminate all "unreasonableness," and in tribute to this ideal of science, on a November morning in 1793, at the height of revolutionary fervor in France, Demoiselle Condeille, "of the opera," ascended the steps of Notre Dame and was crowned "goddess of Reason."[2]

Pierre Bayle had been among the first writers of the period to articulate this new faith. His *Dictionnaire* announced the new scepticism about the old faith as a dogmatic impediment to knowledge. Bayle put religious faith outside of the province of reason and argued that reason must refute all superstitions and dogmas which are, of themselves, inimical to faith. Bayle was not an atheist but a rationalist in the sense that he believed in relying solely on reason's criteria for knowledge and truth while dismissing religion and the merits of any particular confessional distinctions or scriptural interpretations. The Bible is to be believed and obeyed only in so far as its imperatives and teachings are "reasonable" and otherwise dismissed. Bayle's critique of religion and his emphasis on a God revealed in nature, was consistent with Deistic thinking in England which had anticipated the general themes of the Enlightenment; the power of intellect, the insufficiency of faith in the realm of knowledge, the separation of God from His world.

The emphasis on rationalism over theology is met regularly in the Enlightenment but those who proclaimed atheism were not in the mainstream of Enlightenment thought, their message was really for the next century. Helvetius' *De L'Esprit* with its mix of psychology, politics and theory acclaimed one theme, reason. D'Holbach's *Systeme* asserted his principle of materialism and the uselessness of metaphysics. Man, said the Baron, is the sum of his sensations and the mind is a material principle. LaMettrie, theologian turned physician, had already cleared the underbrush of metaphysical detritus. In his *L'Homme Machine* he argued that man is a physio-chemical entity and all of his higher functions are quantitative, related to man's nervous system and changes in its chemical milieu. Cabanis, another physician, was more specific if less aesthetic; the brain thinks its thoughts the way the liver oozes its bile or the kidney its water. Such lessons, uncommon as they may have been in the eighteenth century, were not lost on the nineteenth century when the physio-chemical model was installed as the explanation for man.

These books appearing about mid-century were not so much representative, their materialism was too strong, as they were anticipatory. *The Encyclopedia*, on the other hand, edited by Diderot and D'Alembert, was less materialistic and its contributors did not reject God though they did seem to render Him superfluous. Even the most famous literary name of the age, Voltaire, meant something much different from Leibniz's seventeenth century optimism when he spoke for a world the best of all possible worlds. Voltaire's optimism rested in a belief in man's capacity to create such a world free of the hobgoblins of rigid monarchies, intolerant clerics, and superstitious Christians. Gathered together, and in the company of their ladies of the salon, these lively wits and sharp tongues demolished kings and clerics (even the ·Abbe Raynal joined in), bantered about new economic theories and political movements, and talked of God, but then with circumspection (antireligion was not yet atheism). All the world seemed open to its best possibilities yet. Turgot, himself a positivist, would be moved to remark, "what a crowd of great men on all parts of knowledge, what perfection of human reason."[3]

Etienne Condillac's emphasis on the primacy of sensations in the acquisition of knowledge was a step. Condillac made perception a function of sensation rather than an abstract mental process, giving us a psychology which assigned a diminished role to consciousness-spirit. Condillac's psychology and his views on science and ethics are to be thought of in conjunction with their objects and their utilitarian values, not as ideals or ideas in themselves, a theme repeated in Helvetius' *On the Mind*. Here Helvetius espoused a functional psychology of ethics and morals which treated behavior in relation to passions and instincts, just as it treated intellectual functions in relation to judgement about sense experience without invoking higher motives. Condorcet's sociological optimism also rested on mechanical and sensationalist precepts while Maupertius had suggested a relationship between matter and consciousness in which an animate principle is shared by both; matter is inchoate consciousness. (In the nineteenth century that notion is rejected in favor of its opposite, mind is a derivative of matter). Helvetius' reductive psychology was in line with this, all psychical functions being based on sensation, the foundation for an ethics of utility.

Medical thinking paralleled the shift in the philosophical view occurring during the eithteenth century. Medicine and biology, of course, lend nicely to observation and experiment, indeed medicine moved quickly from being an empirical science in the eighteenth century to an experimental one in the nineteenth. Several eighteenth century "schools," they were not academic bodies, did present medical theories that were evolving along the direction of the mechanistic and deterministic philosophies though none of their physician adherents were in the business of vanquishing religion. The iatrochemists, following VonHelmont, a Capuchin friar, and Francois LeBoe, a physiologist at Leyden, emphasized the physio-chemical bases of body functions such as saliva, bile, digestive juices and the blood in diseases. The iatrochemists felt that medical therapy should be directed to managing the chemical environment of the body, an approach Paracelsus had emphasized in his disputes with the Galenists who relied on herbal cures.

The iatromechanical physicians, on the other hand, viewed the body as a complex machine and disease the result of change in its mechanics and nervous tissues. Friedrich Hoffman and William Cullen, two iconoclasts of the period, emphasized organ tonus, an inherent property of the fibrous organs which allows them to dilate and contract. Hoffman believed that the vital force of the body acts mechanically and that animal spirits are fine material elements which are put in motion through the activity of the soul controlled by the non-material mind. Cullen, the founder of the medical school in Glasgow, related tonus to the energy or forces of the nervous system. These neural concepts of disease, though hardly meant to convey materialistic principles or a philosophy devoid of spirit or soul, were a basis for dogmatic materialism in medicine among physiologists and physicists in the nineteenth century.

Francis Gilsson's theories on irritability in the sixteenth century, expanded by Albrecht VonHaller in the late seventeenth century, had also suggested a materialist position though Haller was a deeply religious and philosophical man. Haller separated the idea of tissue irritability, related to its nervous connections, from sensibility, an inherent property of the tissues themselves. The importance of the work of VonHaller, Hoffman and Cullen for medicine and science lay in its emphasis on treatments directed to physiological derangements rather than on the Hippocratic tradition of reliance on nature. They were physiological physicians, and physiology and pathology would become important sciences in the modern era as the emphasis on the nervous system and the materialistic basis of its function grew.

Clinical medicine was emerging from the shadow of Hippocrates and Galen during this period as well. Padua had become a center for clinical medicine in the sixteenth century with the emphasis on bedside observation, physical diagnosis and classification of symptoms. In the first half of the eighteenth century the center for clinical study shifted to Leyden, where the methods introduced by Francois Leboe, the iatrochemist, were developed by Herman Boerhaave. Boerhaave's influence was felt throughout Europe as his students carried the clinical methods to new centers. VonSwieten and DeHaen went to Vienna, Albrecht VonHaller returned to Bern and Alexander Munro moved to Edinburgh, the first of three Munros to teach there, while later Edinburgh graduates became important figures in medicine in America, Canada and Ireland.

Important parallel developments, both for clinical and research medicine, took place in the new science of pathology. Pathology entered the clinic in the middle of the eighteenth century due mainly to the work of Giambattista Morgagni of Padua. Morgagni followed a long line of distinguished Italian researchers in medicine going back to Alphonse Borelli, the physiologist, who had learned his scientific methods from Galileo. Morgagni was a tireless worker, a meticulous observer and a thorough commentator. He studied pathology for over fifty years, opening cadavers and organs in all phases and conditions of disease and degeneration. He noted the effects wrought by tumors, infections, hemorrhage, trauma and malformation and he correlated these pathologic findings with the clinical information obtained at the bedside. Finally in 1767, at the age of eighty, Morgagni published his monumental treatise in pathologic anatomy *On the Seat and Cause of Disease,* the work which joined the forms of disease in the laboratory with the many faces of disease in the clinic. It was a work very much in the spirit of the age, serving well the methods of science the Enlightenment was championing.

Physiology was also becoming increasingly important as a basic medical science, one with particular relevance to any materialistic philosophy. Men like Volta and Galvani made great advances in the understanding of nervous physiology with the demonstration that muscles and nerves possessed electrical properties, that they, in fact, behaved like non-living things! Medical research in histology, the study of tissue components of various organs, took an important step when Bichat showed that some classes of disease were specific for certain types of tissues with their effects being found on all organs which shared those tissues. This was an important step along the road of reduction in medicine, a shift from general theories or systems in medical thought to the direct observation of "the disease" in its original locus, an approach carried further with cell biology in the nineteenth century and molecular biology in our own time.

French physiology advanced with the same earnestness. Bordeau was among the first to separate glandular function from general physiology by showing that the glands operated autonomously, their activity was separate from mechanical dependency on other organs. Poiseulle studied the behavior and dynamics of fluids, including the blood, and Magendie laid the ground work for research physiology in the nervous system. His pupil, Claude Bernard, assumed the chair in physiology from Magendie and became one of the leaders in European research in the nineteenth century.

Perhaps the leading man in French science at the end of the eighteenth century was Antoinne Lavoisier. Following the experiments of Priestley on "dephlogisted air" and the discoveries by Black and Cavednish, Lavoisier was the one who showed that combustion is the result of the combination of carbon and oxygen. He banished Becher's and Stahl's phlogiston (the idea that burning objects emitted some airy substance, the "phlogiston" and established that respiration is a chemical process, thus helping to answer the old question of heat and anima. These contributions firmly established him as one of the fathers of modern chemistry yet with all of his achievements he remained committed to his religious belief. For that he bowed to the guillotine.

The emergence of science, especially the medical sciences, as a powerful tool for progress and a strong basis for materialistic thinking grew steadily after the Enlightenment and matured with the emphasis on the "Faustian knowledge" of "Force and Matter" (Spengler). Physics and chemistry increasingly removed the last vestiges of vitalism from medicine and biology and the nascent materialism in iatrochemical and iatromechanical medical theories matured with the prodigious work in the basic sciences. Advances in brain and nervous system physiology, especially the demonstration of the electrical properties of tissues, suggested a link between living things and physical forces, a notion which became a basic scientific principle in the nineteenth century laboratory. After the work of Harvey and Lavoisier the circulation of the blood and respiration were increasingly viewed as mechanical functions in a body essentially a machine and the physiological advances of the nineteenth century would validate this. Man was being reduced to his composite physio-chemical systems following Maupertius' law of least action, Maier's conservation of energy and Carnot's entropy. The concepts of work, force and energy, all derivatives of the principle of matter, were applied to the physiology of man. The result was a scientific structure which was deterministic and mechanistic; physio-chemical processes are integrated and self-executing. Thus, in medicine beyond all other sciences, the new man was taking shape, he was becoming man without soul.

Nineteenth century advances in physics, the understanding that light emits as waves rather than corpuscles (as Newton held), the connection between electricity and magnetism and their conformity to the same mathematics as gravity, and atomic theory with its planetary analogy seemed to give incontrovertible evidence of the principle of mechanism in nature and cosmos. Mechanism and process were viewed as immediate and immanent properties of nature without any relation to teleology and first cause. After all, does not the idea that energy is neither created nor destroyed say something quite final as regards ultimate causality? (It was Maupertius' recognition of such a conclusion in Descartes' notion of conservation of energy that led him to his theory of least action, thereby keeping God in the equation).

In the nineteenth century medicine, once again, stood out, especially research physiology and biochemistry. For one, both medicine and biology lent themselves splendidly to reductive and experimental methods. Secondly, Newton seemed to have put the cosmos in good order so that medicine appeared to offer the best possibility for another Newton (as it would after the bomb in the twentieth century). At the same time it naturally fell to medicine and biology to probe the old questions; the mind-body problem and the material bases for life. Medicine, as it explored these issues, seemed to provide further justification for throwing out God. The success of the materialist approaches in the medical laboratory were then joined to the religious scepticism of the philosophers of the nineteenth century.

The Enlightenment materialists, beginning with Bayle and including D'Holbach, Helvetius, Cabanis and LaMettrie, had written from a sense of future development rather than from evidence at hand but within a few decades the situation changed substantially. The nineteenth century philosophers of materialism had the growing evidence of science, and this was a strong challenge to religion and the old dogma. The materialist philosophers could be increasingly bold and emphatic because of science; man is the new God and man will know this god through science. Man no longer needs to invoke spiritual forces outside himself, all begins and ends in man, the final achievement of matter and material existence. The high priest of this thinking, Ludwig Feuerbach, was in the line of direct descent from the materialists of the Enlightenment but he added the final verse to their song of reason. He wrote; "God was my first thought [he studied for the ministry], Reason my second, and man my third and last [thought]."[4]

Feuerbach had studied Hegel and attended his lectures in Berlin. Hegel had taught that "absolute spirit" was an idea realized in thought and perfected through the dialectic of history (personal and spiritual). Hegel's view was essentially a pantheistic philosophy in so far as the Absolute pervades everything. Feuerbach, however, returned thought to its origin in man and nature while viewing thought as an organic activity arising from matter. Feuerbach's etiology of religion was closely related to this in that he made religion the thought projection of the ego. The God-idea is the projection of man's own essence into spirit, while his relation to nature is the origin of religious worship. Feuerbach believed that man had to rid himself of the God fantasy and recognize the psychological truth of religious thinking (its basis in cosmic fear) so that he can concern himself with man. In this scheme theology is a transitional formulation, anthropology is the final one. Feuerbach's psychology of religion anticipated much of Freud's while his materialism (matter is real, man is functional matter) was in keeping with a growing body of medical evidence.

Feuerbach's philosophy was shared by other young Hegelians, Bruno Bauer, Arnold Ruge and David Strauss. Strauss, earlier than Feuerbach, had emphasized the importance of demythologizing religion. He felt that all of the attributes imputed to Christ could not have been realized in one man but only in humanity. Strauss was preaching a universal ideal of humanity. The parallels between Strauss' system and Comtean thought are striking, Comte's "great being," humanity, is the same as Strauss' while Feuerbach's and Comte's historical stages, religion (superstition), philosophy, positive knowledge are identical to those in Feuerbach's personal odyssey.

Scientific advances went hand in hand with this new outlook and were most impressive in the medical laboratory; the pathologic anatomy of Morgagni gradually passed into the histology of Malphigi and Bichat, then to the cell biology of Schleiden, Schwann and Virchow. Humoral principles in pathologic anatomy was last held by Roditansky, in Virchow's cellular pathology humoral theory is gone and the cell is the unit of disease and cell physiology is the mechanism. Vitalism is banished after Claude Bernard finished the work of Magendie with the principle that specific organs possess specific functions. These developments did not translate into absolute materialism for those who advanced them but for others this kind of evidence could mean little else.

The medical scientists Ludwig Buechner, Carl Vogt and Jacob Moleschott were unequivocal materialists. For them the properties of matter were the source and extent of all knowledge. Buechner sought "everywhere a natural and law-determined connection of all phenomena of the world."[5] His search would proceed no further than matter because nothing else exists. Mole-schott's sentiments were similar, he depicted life forces as the result of "interacting and interweaving physical and chemical forces."[6] For Carl Vogt it is just this, the brain oozes its ideas just like organs ooze their juices (recall Cabanis).

The work of Karl Woehler had lent impetus to Vogt's pronouncement. In 1828 Woehler was able to synthesize urea, demonstrating that a "life" chemical, thought possible only within the living organism, could be assembled in the laboratory. Johannes Muller's work on nervous function was leading to a similar conception. Muller was able to demonstrate that different sense organs respond to specific stimuli with their own particular sensation. Sensation is not a general phenomena referrable to vital forces but is the result of specific physiological and anatomical connections. Muller influenced a generation of researchers including Virchow, Schwann and Henle in cell studies and Herman Helmholtz, Ernest Brucke, Carl Ludwig and Emil DuBois-Reymond in physics, physiology and anatomy. Helmholtz's "school" was committed to explaining all life processes through physio-chemical equations. Helmholtz studied nervous physiology and determined the velocity of nerve impulses. He made important contributions in optics, in research in electricity and in theoretical physics. Helmholtz was a committed empiricist and his devotion to method as well as his achievements made him a giant of the period and one of his pupils, Brucke, later taught a promising young student those methods in his neurophysiology laboratory. The student was Sigmund Freud.

Virchow's cell biology was one of the great advances of nineteenth century medicine. Virchow was able to demonstrate that it is at the cell level where disease processes take their origin. Virchow had become interested in the microscopic study of pathologic specimens under Johanne Muller. Cellular pathology, of course, was strong evidence against the old humoral concepts and the general theories of "dyscrasia" which held sway through the time of Karl Rokitansky, a giant in pathological anatomy in Vienna who had continued in the tradition of Morgagni in this important medical science.

Pathological anatomy, in fact, had helped displace humoral theories a century earlier and was one of the first medical disciplines to bridge the gap between bedside and laboratory medicine. Significantly, both gross anatomy and pathological anatomy were revealing more details regarding brain function. Brain topography revealed that different anatomical areas not only controlled particular body functions but were involved in intellectual and affective life as well (e.g. the research of Flourens on the cerebral hemispheres). The isolation of the reflex arc, demonstrating that man responds to sudden and potent stimuli just as other animals, unconsciously, was a step. The discovery that various glands secrete under the influence of nerve impulses was another, leading to the idea that physiological "reflexes" could be trained or conditioned by associative techniques (e.g. Pavlov). Thus, neural physiology and experimental psychology were complementing each other in the use of association techniques and stimuli-response testing, while inching their way toward the mainstream of medical thought at the turn of the century. There was an obvious lesson; Mind and brain are subject to the same physical determinants as is the animal body, one of the profound "facts" to issue from the medical research laboratory.

The greatest medical physiologist of the century, Claude Bernard, worked tirelessly to separate experiment and life processes from any spiritual or vital forces. Bernard wanted to show that vitalism does not have a place in the study of life processes or in our knowledge of man.

> I think that every phenomenon called vital must sooner or later be reduced to definite properties of organized or organic matter. We may, of course, use words like vitality as chemists use affinity or physicists force but when the conditions necessary to phenomenon are known then occult forces will disappear![7]

One can hardly fail to recall Newton's same concern in physics:

> Principles (gravity, magnetism, etc.) I consider not as occult qualities... but as general laws of nature... their truth appearing to us by phenomena. To derive two or three general principles of motion from phenomena... would be a great step though the causes of those principles are not yet discovered. Therefore I scruple not to propose the principles of motion and leave their causes to be found out.[8]

Newton would say that "to tell us that every thing is endowed with an quality by which it acts and produces manifest effects is to tell us nothing."[9]

Bernard also recognized the role of accidental observation in the genesis of a theory and the formulation of a hypothesis to be tested by the experiment, as well as the building of a theory and the elaboration of a general law from the facts. Nonetheless, it was the fact which was supreme for Bernard:

> In the presence of a well noted new fact which contradicts a theory, instead of keeping the theory and abandoning the fact, I should keep and study the fact and hasten to give up the theory.

In that regard Bernard is the very model of the cautious experimenter whose interest is in the process being observed, its reproducibility and its predictability. That is the essence of the new knowledge. Science is reductive-controlling knowledge. It describes nature's next move and moves to manipulate it; the desideratum in clinical and research medicine. In Bernard's nineteenth century method, as in ours, the fact dominates all knowledge. The facts, of course, remove all spiritual categories, and are the only certainty, and science is the only way of getting the facts. Yet Bernard sensed a limitation in limiting everything to the facts of the experiment:

> It is as if there existed a preestablished design of each organism...though considered separately, each physiological process...reveals a special bond and seems directed by some invisible guide."[11]

If the harmony of the whole seemed obvious in physiology (as in cosmology) then something must be the informing principle of that harmony. Either the body, like the cosmos, is impelled by an inner necessity (matter is itself a principle of harmony) or the mysterious notion of design in biology must have something to do with Voltaire's "clockmaker," hence was part of the "God problem," and the problem of the forces of the cosmos and in life remained occult. The surgeon Gerdy once replied to a conclusion Bernard held regarding the findings of a particular experiment, "whenever life enters into phenomena conditions may be as similar as we please, the results may still be different."[12] And Osler reminds us of that special problem in medicine "there are no diseases, only patients," something other than mechanism is working here.

Nineteenth century medical sciences marched on the facts nonetheless. Nineteenth century physics dealt with forces at a distance, dynamic force, a heritage from Newton after Aristotle's statics had been vanquished by Galileo's simple forces of contact. Physics also searched for the principle(s) which would banish all possibilities for occultism and even though the concepts in physical science remained mysterious physicists sought to define them as "laws" of matter, issuing from the activity of matter in the physical world and in the cosmos.

Medical scientists sought to write biology in much the same way, and the idea of scientific law, inevitable and inviolable, took over the new social sciences as well. Thus the theories of evolution (Darwin) and the unconscious (Freud) would ultimately rest in the materialist principle, as would the most conspicuous social theory of the nineteenth century (Marx). In each of these force and determinism replaced spirit and overtook the idea of the individual with the idea of man, man's animal origins, his unconscious motives and his sociological evolution. In the theories of Freud, Marx and Darwin there could be no room for spirit because man was fulfilling "the law" in his material condition. From here on the only place one could hear the word "spirit" spoken without jest would be in church litany or ghost stories.

The Twentieth Century

Nietzsche left us on a steamy summer day in 1900, by most accounts insane and Godless. Nietzsche, after all, kept telling us that God is dead, we had killed Him. He may well have added that it was science that presided at the interment. Science was now tightening its grip with startling swiftness. The Quantum Age was at hand, the physical sciences were increasing domination over the physical world, and biology and medicine were revolutionizing man's self image, even suggesting a scientific theory of the soul. Biology, of course, was already enamored with evolution theory which influenced a new view of the psyche.

Philosophy was congenial; positivism and materialism were inspiring the developing social sciences and the medical revolution which was wiping away the last vestiges of spirit and vital forces. At the same time the successes of the research laboratory and new technologies were feeding the philosophical view. Science and philosophy, then, were symbiotic but this really meant the eclipse of traditional philosophy and, certainly, the withering of the old metaphysics.

Nineteenth century philosophers such as Feuerbach and Marx had spoken in megahistorical terms derived from the more spiritual Hegel while others, like St. Simon and Comte, embraced an intellectual positivism which was the ultimate expression of the thought of Condorcet, Condillac, Helvetius and D'Holbach. Common to all of the materialist-positivist writings, however, was the idea of the practical absurdity of the former preoccupation with God and Spirit. They offered a new religion, the religion of mankind, such as Comte envisioned when he preached about "the great being—humanity...the only solution to the problem of man."[1]

Science was the obvious vehicle to advance the "great being." What else could so powerfully assert man's control over those unseen forces that his ancestors once hid from in caves? Biology and medicine could show us what man is, other "sciences" would tell us why he does what he does, others how he does what he does, and still other sciences would help make sure that he does what he should—all in the name of mankind! The key to the widespread acceptance of Marx, Darwin, and Freud was their idea of that mythical entity, mankind. The individual could disagree with the ultimate meaning of economic or zoological man or with psychic evolution, but it would be no contest against the mega-theories of Marxist sociology, Darwinian evolution and Freudian psychology, forces with an organic life of their own.

Developments in the physical and chemical science, advances in biology and medicine and the ever widening scope of physics and astronomy were intimately related to the radical change in thought now taking place. From here on all subjects would be studied by scientific methods, either they would become weighing and measuring disciplines or become counterfeit. All knowledge must in some measure issue through the scientific mode to hold any value in the market place of ideas. Knowledge of man himself was included so that the study of the behavior and motives of groups would be an extension of the methods of study of the individual in the medical laboratory. Social physiology and social physics could contribute only by following zoology and physiology. Medicine and biology were paradigmatic, social theory should seek to model itself the way the physiocrats once meant economics to follow physiology. It was in biology and medicine, moreover, that the materialistic view would be most persuasive. Biology and medicine offered two great theories for this twentieth century world view, psychoanalytic theory and evolution. Whatever the scientific merits of psychoanalysis and evolution (they are still debated) both have had a profound effect on modern life in the West. It may be said that by exposing the "subconscious fraud" in religious thinking they have heightened modern man's self-alienation and loss of meaning.

Both theories had a tremendous impact on the directions and practice of medicine, removing it from an ancient and venerable heritage in the service of the whole man, the spiritual man who is just incidentally a "sick man." Medicine was always closely bound to religion because both kept that special vigil against death and could not therefore dismiss the sick man's greater spiritual need. By the beginning of the century it was already done, medicine became committed to the scientific ideal, forfeiting its special claim on behalf of the spiritual man. It was psychoanalysis, ironically, the medical "soul science," which helped medicine on that unhappy course.

The appearance of psychoanalysis was a watershed. Certainly psychoanalysis did not mark the beginning of man's interest in the life of the mind or in theories of the unconscious, but it did suggest that they could be made scientific by basing them on an archeology of mind and the confluence of psychic forces common to all men. Even though the audience was limited at first the message spread in influence as its theoretic flaws were overlooked by a world impatient for new knowledge about man. Psychoanalysis, after all, offered the possibility for understanding human actions beyond even the loftiest speculations of men of letters or philosophy.

Curiosity about mental illness and physical afflictions is as old as medicine. Madness, alterations of the elements or humors, was recorded in the literature of the Greeks and discussed by their philosophers. In the medieval and early modern period the relation between physical debility and mental instability, especially melancholia and mania, occupied a considerable literature and in much of that intellectual tradition also suggested mystical, spiritual and demonic forces, even as it did for primitives, and was closely bound to the concept of sin. The notion that mental disease had an explanation in the subconscious separate from sin, physical debility and conscious activity, however, took form with the work of Sigmund Freud.

Psychoanalysis became a medical specialty after Freud discarded traditional considerations of hysteria and conversion reactions in favor of the premise that hysteria was a psychological problem rather than a neuroanatomic one. Freud joined this insight to an appropriate therapeutic, the analysis or exploration of the psychic residues of the subject's life experiences. Freud's method used the logotherapy of free association, his "chimney sweep," an advance over earlier hypnotic methods such as those in vogue at Paris during Freud's stay with M. Charcot. Freud's work was the beginning of the development of psychoanalysis and the gradual unfolding of general theories of psychic and social life. Freud was on his way to making psychoanalysis a genuine "geisteswissenschaften," a medical soul science for the twentieth century.

Freud presented a formal theory of the subconscious within the framework of the prevailing scientific models of the time, suggesting that the psyche had a specific topography analogous to the neuroanatomic model and specific activities akin to measurable forces. This is no surprise when one considers that Freud was thoroughly familiar with the methods of quantitative research in the basic medical sciences. He had established himself as a good worker in the physiology laboratory of Ernst Brucke and as a careful student of neurology under Theodore Meynert and Jean Charcot. His physiological research was in the tradition of the school of Helmholtz and DuBois-Reymond with its emphasis on mechanism and the actions and properties of matter and the forces of attraction and repulsion. Freud added another dimension, however, an "archeology" of the psyche. Freud was greatly influenced by the evolutionary views of Charles Darwin and he incorporated Darwin's phylogenetic theory into his own idea of the ontogeny of psychic processes, using the evolutionary model to explain the genesis of psychopathology. But that introduced a disturbing contradiction.

Freud, careful and exacting experimenter, based his theories on such unsupportable propositions as an historically presumed murder of a tribal father at the hands of his sons, and the subsequent appearance of totem phenomena and the incest taboos as a recollection of and expiation for this original parricide. He also linked these to his theory of the Oedipal conflict which he developed after a lengthy self-analysis precipitated by his father's death, while arriving at the hidden significance of dreams through a thorough analysis of his own. Finally, he colored the data of his analyses with his own projections, imputing feelings of his own to the patients he studied. All of these elements made psychoanalysis a compelling personal vision, indeed, but hardly valid science.

Psychoanalysis kept the appearance of science, however, by using the vocabulary of contemporary German physics, terms such as force, reaction, outflow, discharge etc., as well as by complying with the analytical and deductive methods of medical science as exhibited in the developments in physio-chemical and cellular pathology of the time. Psychoanalysis was, in a sense, the last of the medical macro-theories to be put forth before the biochemical and molecular sciences finally vanquished all general medical theories in favor of reductive analysis. After psychoanalysis, medical thinking magnified its measuring sticks and severly narrowed their objects so that life processes were studied on an ever decreasing scale, increasingly removed from their condition within the harmony of an organic whole.

Psychoanalysis was also different. The psyche is not a demonstrable entity in the usual sense of the term nor are psychic forces simple physical forces, the psyche is no mere "place" or "activity." Its activities or functions may have been topographically demarcated (id, ego, superego) by Freud but therapeutically this has no relevance because psychotherapy could not be effectively "administered" as if one were treating a traditional illness or pathological state. But there was another way in which psychoanalysis was different from earlier medical theories, it was also the basis for social theory.

As Freud's thinking progressed he came to view psychoanalysis as a way of explaining the evolution and dynamics of culture. His theories on instincts, repression, guilt and sublimation formed the basis for a theory of social life and society. Freud believed that the instincts are the primary motive forces in human life and that the individual only arrives at an equilibrium between the beast within and the world outside because of the demand of the superego and the reality principle. These place the individual in a conflict producing state; he must repress his instinctual life and individual desires for the sake of social integration but this repression, according to Freud, produced the conditions for mental illness. Likewise, the resulting conflicts feed the potential for the ills of civilization because the socialization process gives us particular men who find a place, if you will, through an uneasy truce with the demands of social membership and denial of the instincts. This results in a new level of anxiety and leads to all of the excesses of culture-man, destructive of those very foundations which were to direct the efforts of superego in its integrative work. Freud thought that man could not help himself in this destructiveness, it is the price he pays for the repression of his instincts. Antisocial behavior issues from nature-man shedding his skin sociologically.

There is another side to this. Any emotional transaction would be a psychological deal, the investment of the superego yielding a specific dividend, the possibility for living socially, but it is a deal, not a matter of freedom or moral choice. The transaction is rooted in conflict and repression and the uncertainty of our motives; no moral choice here, only utilitarian preferences managed by the superego. Freud could not admit that the "essential" transactions issue from spirit man, not so much at war with himself as in search of meaning from within, that was just too much existential freedom for Freud. Freud emphasized the war but the war had an old history, it was precisely such Manicheanism that Christianity rejected early on. Man was already rehabilitated when Freud arrived, Freud made him a patient again.

Freud could not really find a way to lift us out of our psychological chains. He made instincts, drives and complexes more powerful agents in human behavior than conscience, free will and spirit. Freud's theory essentially finds us bound by the calculations of the agent of right action he calls the superego, that part of the psyche which guides our choices and facilitates our socialization. The problem with the superego, however, is that it is an infantile "organ," really no more than a primitive censor which guards against the excesses of the biological man. Our Judeo-Christian heritage, on the other hand, teaches that each man possesses a conscience which is provident of his whole being, while in harmony with the natural law, and not just the conditions of nature. Conscience doesn't merely arbitrate the right pragmatic choice, superego does that, conscience informs man about the morality of choosing. It tells him that he is free to respond as a biological man, reflexively, and he is also free to deliberate on his choice and act on his ideal...the privilege of choosing is his.

Conscience is a positive movement, the ego to the other. Superego is self-directed, its relationship to the world is utilitarian as the arbiter of right action which tends to the demands of the "reality principle." Freud argued that the individual becomes socialized when the superego instructs the id (the psychic dwelling place of the instincts and drives) and he believed that the superego was the author of the "laws" of society and social living. This view confuses the heirarchy of values. The superego may teach but it does not legislate. The ideals, traditions and beliefs of a society are the primary values, they are in place before the superego; they are the rules, and each man must learn them to live fully as a man. Let's say it another way, civilization and social life is founded in a normative world of natural and Divine Law. Conscience guards the gates and informs all men of moral choice in that world.

There is another difficulty with this business of the superego. If we accept Freud's formulation about social life and human motives, id constantly lurks just beneath the social man and individual actions cannot really be viewed as defects in the moral man. Evil then comes only to represent the psychic defect in all men and the result of forces that man cannot really control. Religion, of course, rejects this. Religion says that we are not bound by the dynamics of the subconscious, we are instead free to choose. We must recall the hubris of Lear, the faint-heartedness of MacBeth and that special melancholy of Hamlet. Here action was met with consequences that were inevitable because of a moral defect in the man. The fault was their own because in a condition of "fallenness" men can choose not to choose, or can choose to embrace evil. Freud's psychanalysis and religion mark their positions clearly, either we cannot help what we are because we are only animals, or we are as much as we choose to be because we are much more.

There may well be a subconscious and it was part of Freud's genius to seek it but it's part of his failure that he overestimated its power while limiting its expression. Analysis, in the search for the significant in the subconscious and a reconciliation between subconscious and conscious, provides therapeutic possibilities but this is hardly an endeavor meant to discover meaning. Therapy allows the psyche to reach an accomodation with the individual's existential condition, giving him more psychic energy to go on, without really telling him why he should!

The subconscious keeps some dark secrets, man struggles with eros in bizarre ways, he dances with thanatos, his drives and instincts are all part of the biological man. Freud's mistake was to rest his case about man here, but it was a mistake that was inevitable once religion was rejected. Freud didn't really reject religion, the subconscious need, he rejected religion, the conscious belief. He believed that the origin of religious thinking was an expression of psychic dependency tied to a deeply rooted need to mitigate cosmic fear. Freud meant psychoanalysis to rid the subconscious of that hobgoblin, reassuring us that there is nothing beyond or above man, so there is nothing to fear. The individual must reconcile himself to the reality of this existential aloneness. Psychoanalysis, he promised, would get us there.

Freud's denial of religion is the heart of the matter. Psychoanalysis, no doubt, has been a modality for helping man realize the condition of his nature-life, but without helping him in his quest for meaning. The "chimney sweep" is preeminently a method for adjusting the present by invoking the past while religion is far less concerned with any archeology of the mind. The religious experience is essentially a confrontation with the self which is hopeful for the future, and not only a future beyond death but a future actualizing in the present. Freud, however, wanted psychoanalysis to set man free from what he believed was a repressive and compelling religious structure which he thought was a force in much of the dark side of history. Freud believed that his new science would allow individuals, and society, to accept the finality of death and the absence of the spiritual force in life with equanimity. He could not offer that hope which Nietzsche once remarked cynically, but correctly, "is a much stronger stimulant to life than any single instance of happiness that may occur."[3] Yet Freud expected psychoanalysis to be greeted with enthusiasm as religion withdrew, even if it could only replace hope with "reality."

One might ask why religion, which offers hope, can be called repressive while a pessimistic psychology can serve as a basis for optimism. Certainly religion doesn't dispute the claims of psychoanalysis or biology about man in his natural state, including his profound anxiety. Man is a little bit of everything everyone says about him, religion bases its own legitimacy on that evidence. But if religion did not summon man to something more, then religion would be no different from any materialistic psychology or philosophy. It is precisely because religion recognizes the spiritual need and man's freedom to satisfy such a deeply felt need that it is the only human experience which can serve as the basis for a genuine optimism. This was one of the points which led to an historic break in the early years of psychoanalysis.

Carl Jung of Zurich seemed the logical heir to Freud in the psychoanalytic community, very European, widely read and Aryan. Jung was Freud's choice and they got on at the beginning but Freud's dogmatism became a problem for Jung as time passed. Freud's theoretic structure and approaches to therapy were rigid systems, and Freud held to them all the more as others developed their own views. Jung, on the other hand, could not accept the structure, not the sexual theory and the Oedipus complex, not the absence of spiritual meaning, not the rigidity of the therapeutic dialogue. Jung's view was wider, more open, more mystical. He had a great interest in the complex and mysterious business of primitive mythology, alchemical metaphysics, and the problem of language and symbols, all of which played heavily in the development of his theories.

Jung, like Freud, reconstituted the psyche archeologically but he was much more impressionistic. He believed that all psychic significations could ultimately be traced to archetypes, primordial symbols which represent the oldest and most basic ideas that dwell in the unconscious. Jung saw these archetypes as the key to elucidating the secret truths of the psyche which he believed were fundamentally religious and spiritual. Dreams, he felt, were a particularly fruitful area for explication as dream content, thematic dreams, could best be understood in relation to the archetypes, the universal and timeless symbols of man in search of meaning. Jung also believed that myths were collective memory records of real events and that the language and symbols of the myth overlay a profound story which touched the truth of the collective experience conveyed in the myth. Jung felt that the search for truth is related to unraveling the meaning of the symbols, the deeper layer of meaning, hidden in the various manifestations of the archetypes.

Freud's view was more rigid and deterministic, the unconscious meanings are zoological. They may represent events that Freud thought had a real history, alright, but they are of no use in bringing a new synthesis, rather are the essential stuff of neuroses. Freud believed that the psyche passes through the phylogenetic history of the race as well as through various stages on its way to maturity in the individual and that both are particularly charged with repressive material and the stuff of neuroses. These fix, if you will, an iron law of the unconscious by which the unconscious is bound to the instinctual and whose conscious expression is at bottom pathologic. Jung, on the other hand, though recognizing a phylogenetic matrix in the unconscious saw the imprint of its symbols less as the material of psychopathology and more as the shared experience of man in search of meaning; true enough, sometimes this matrix is a basis for pathology but more often it is the impetus to self-discovery and realization of his greatest needs. Obviously, these considerations colored both men's sense of therapy. Freud saw it as a tool for getting the psyche in harmony with the demands of social and cultural life (even while he saw their repressive nature as a cause of pathology). For Freud therapy was "life-adjustment." This, in effect, says you are sick because every man is sick but you must still function in the milieu in which you find yourself. Don't ask about the meaning much less why you are here at all, get on with living. Jung recognized the insufficiency of that therapeutic goal, more is needed than just getting on, there must be a reason for doing so. Jung believed that therapy would help man realize that his life has meaning and each man can find this within himself. Therapy was the tool, meaning the end, "individuation" the process—the process of recognizing the self which would answer the question of meaning for him who would ask.

Jung saw the danger in the analyst imposing his system on his patient. He emphasized the necessity for empathetic therapy, in the old sense of the term, wherein the therapist finds meaning along with his patient. In so far as every man is seeking the same thing, this is the other side of "individuation." The issue was the possibilities for the patient speaking openly and being heard as a "fellow man," not just as a patient. This concern was also evident among many who were not professional analysts. The Existential philosopher and Jewish spiritual leader, Martin Buber, saw this as the guiding principle of therapy. Hence, Buber would remind us that the analytic encounter must be a true "I-thou" meeting

> what is demanded of him [the therapist] is that he draw the particular case out of the covert methodological objectification and himself step forth out of the role of professional superiority into the elementary situation between one who calls and one who is called...in a decisive hour he [and the patient] has left the closed room of psychology and stepped into the air where self is exposed to self."[5]

The therapist is the guide in this psychic exploration and follows all its paths. The patient will follow only if the right path is cleared, but he will turn away if some paths are open only to the guide and others are closed by him. The therapist must lead the patient precisely by being unconditionally open to him, so that the patient can emerge freely. Having discovered together a path then it is always the patient, alone, who chooses to lead himself through. In a very real sense there is no way, one finds the way by going.

The great tragedy of psychoanalysis, of course, has been its refusal to call the spiritual man. The technician of the psyche, the therapist, has been preoccupied with pathology rather than existence, with the unfortunate result that the patient has usually mistaken the insufficiency of analysis for the absence of meaning. Patients no longer seek meaning but therapy for accomodation, so called "life adjustment." That might be necessary and appropriate but it is clearly limited since the symptoms requiring accomodation therapy are only heralds of the disease. The disease, of course, is bound to the problem of meaning. Once the therapist, and so the patient, see that the problem of meaning is a far bigger thing than the management of pathology, then psychotherapy can become a tool for realization, the real cure.

There is really no choice between therapy for accomodation and therapy for meaning, the former ultimately demands the latter. The patient, "in the clearing and illuminating open space of being," can summon his spiritual self and discover the meaning of his predicament. Language, of course, grants this possibility, "it brings about the original interwovenness of man and things in the world and this can come only if and as long as those who are interwoven are really there and come to light with regard to one another."⁶ For the sick man and his doctor it is not only the words but how they are heard. Words can conceal or reveal so that what is spoken must then be measured against what is meant, and what is left unspoken must be weighed against what that silence meant to say.

The therapeutic word is essential to this discovery, to the realization that, as Buber says, "no human encounter lacks a hidden significance." Psychoanalysis holds out the possibility for this and for the prospect for self-realization but it must disentangle itself from all systems and schools and interrogate the whole man. Jung recognized the importance of putting away typologies in treatment. "Practical medicine," he said, "is an art, as is practical analysis...learn theories but put them aside when you touch the miracle of the living soul. The patient is there to be treated and not to verify a theory."⁷ For this to happen, for the patient to really be helped, the dialogue must unconditionally open. Only a dialogue between the sick man and the physician which is truly reciprocal, each knowing that when he speaks, as Siirala says, "he is never a mere individual, he is always a fellow man as well,"⁸ can bring healing. If disease, psychological or somatic, is not merely a disturbance in the autonomy of an organ or the action of a "complex" or a "germ" but might be an appeal to self or community, then the word becomes decisive in the explication. It opens to the truth of Jung's belief that, "The object of therapy is not the neurosis (illness) but the man who waits...it comes from the totality of a man's life from his psychic experiences within the family or even the social group."⁹

Unhappily, now, the real healing value of words is lost in the modern notion of the placebo, which has come to stand only for some element (physical, chemical or verbal) which realizes an outcome independent of scientifically explainable principles. Scientific medicine employs the placebo in a formal methodology which measures the impact of a neutral factor against a "specific" one while efforts are made to eliminate suggestibility, persuasion and the talking cure, the very elements which are primary forces in healing.

Historically, "placebo thinking," the idea of the curative power of words, was linked to the unseen forces in illness and had little to do with method excepting perhaps as different beliefs organized the rituals of healing. These beliefs were of two kinds, the belief a particular culture held about the mysteries of life (therefore illness and death) and the sick man's personal beliefs. The healing ritual itself introduced a third element which was constitutive of the healing, the trust the sick man had in the mediator between his own condition and the mysterious. Somewhere in the complexity of these elements lies the hidden dynamic of the placebo idea and its power for self-validation. The key figure is the sick man for it is his belief in what is held out to him, by its being true for him, that he might recover. The word is the centerpiece in this phenomenology because it is the way in which belief is extended and the cure made manifest. If the unique element in human life is language and the projection of being into the world, then the soul is the object of the curing word and the soul must be in its correct mode of acceptance, what the Greeks called "parachesis." Then healing can occur and the soul restored to "sophrosyne," or internal harmony, such as Plato and the Greeks recognized.

The placebo idea, in the old understanding, still counts in our medicine because the word still matters to the sick man. The therapeutic word still can overcome the cultural falling away from faith even as it can overcome each man's doubt because of each man's hope. Certainly, this applies to the sick man, and it applies to political man as well in a social world conditioned to believe in words spoken to heal social ills. Plato said that they are the decisive element in the political sphere, the tool of the politician who works by persuasion, so that even in our own day there is no society without its great "social placebos." Thus Simone Weil could rightly remark "Though we live in an age... far removed from the prelogical condition, it is still certain that we believe in the magic efficacy of words far more than any savage ever did."

Contemporary psychiatry still uses the talking cure but it is virtually absent from the rest of medicine which views the talking cure with contempt because it is unscientific. Modern medicine seeks objectivity in diagnoses and treatment, the kind of objectivity, in fact, the Hippocratics said proved the efficacy of their own methods—they even worked in the unbelieving! This modern obsession with objectivity has overtaken psychiatry to the point that a whole new view of psychic life is emerging.

Neurobiology is concerned with the physical and chemical aspects of "mind" suggesting mechanistic models in the way physical sciences mean the term; thoughts, emotions, feelings are the manifestations of physio-chemical events, expressions of the "discharge" of millions of chemical connections among countless nerve foci. This neurobiologic model reduces all conscious and subconscious life to the level of matter and its physiochemical interactions, a radical interpretation of man which will vanquish the idea of spirit and free will. Older psychoanalytic and psychiatric theories, remember, still allowed a spiritual (non-material) dimension because of the mythic nature of pathogenesis (Freud) or the struggle for meaning (Jung). The recollection of parricide, the dynamics of the complexes and the wide ranging eros and thanatos were not physiological, so that even for Freud psychic life was not to be understood wholly by crude physicalism. In that sense his psychoanalysis was an atypical science, its hypotheses were non-quantifiable, and not strictly in line with the reductive, measuring method of physics and chemistry even though it borrowed their concepts and methods. Nonetheless, once medical science removed spirit and mythos from the clinic the next step was to remove it from the couch.

The advances in neurobiology, and in molecular medicine, including genetics, and the application of quantum theory to biology have brought psychiatry and analysis to the point where they will soon remove spirit and free will from any independent ontological position. The new neurochemical definitions of mind and psyche will be much harder to refute precisely because they come by way of weighing and measuring science. The old psychiatry, after all, was always vulnerable to the charge that it was insufficiently rigorous, long on hypotheses and short on "proofs." The neurochemical model suffers no such disadvantage because it is no longer dealing with the psyche as previously conceived. Mental illness is now understood with specific reference to genetical and biochemical models (something Freud had predicted). Today we simply try to say that neurophysiological derangements are the trouble with the troubled. Now the therapy of mind takes on a whole new thrust, not in need of the individual's participation, only his submission. The freedom possible in the talking cure is gone because it is unnecessary that the subject even recognize his infirmity, much less accede to some meddling with it. All that is required now is that the remedy have the same objectification as the defect.

The fact that previous analytic theory kept to psychic (non-material) references still preserved the possibilities for psychic healing. Mental illness did not occupy a physical space, it was not a disease of brain tissue, per se, (that insight was the great advance of psychoanalysis) so that for it to successfully play out a complex process of interiorization was necessary. The subconscious had to be penetrated by freedom. Molecular determinism, on the other hand, describes mental disease in terms of fixed physio-chemical events. The consequence of these directions in the new biology and in the entire medical enterprise in the closing days of the twentieth century is the technical reality of bioengineering. Now both psychoanalysis and sin are being eliminated because the psyche can be reconstituted to fit a new therapeutic ideal defined by the scientific elite. Biochemical tailoring presents the greatest possibilities yet imagined for power over man and nature, even a therapeutic for the entire polity, for it is simple enough to move from traditional medical goals to sociological ones. For the first time man really can contemplate remaking himself to his own image. By that I mean he can direct his technology to removing "undesirable" physical, psychological, and social traits in the interest of the community, even if it means treating all the members! Genetic engineering already has a demonstrated capacity in bacteriology and virology. The technical apparatus is in place, the skillful manipulation of genetic material is a reality. The prospects for radically reordering the incidence of infectious disease, antibiotic resistance and viral oncogenesis by additions and deletions in the DNA code and/or the replication process are matters for practical consideration now. At the same time many breakthroughs have occured in the identification of neurochemical systems which play a part in modulating mood and behavior, sleep and dreams, various circadian rhythms, even aesthetic and cognitive sensibilities. The introduction of precursor molecules or analogs either through dietary or drug interventions or similar manipulations of permissive and/or inhibitory systems affords us the potential to modify many aspects of neurophysiological function and control the molecular and humoral inputs to psychological activity.

Never before has man been in possession of the knowhow to alter specific higher functions. We are not, after all, tampering with accidental properties of nature, now we are talking about remaking nature from our blueprints. Are we on the threshold of producing social and political compliance, tailoring human beings to specific tasks in the name of polity? Will the therapeutic-controlling urge finally produce a man no longer responsible because he is managed? Is this management less iniquitous precisely because it is molecular and not "psychological?" Will we allow the march of science and the biology of mind to mean that we can no longer charge man with a moral obligation? If conscious life takes place in a chemical crucible, is hostile and violent behavior only some wild alchemy which arranges itself? With this alchemy how can we hold people responsible for their actions, their evil or their genius? Evil becomes a neurophysiological category. It is all molecular? Not only is man no longer a moral agent, he isn't even subject to passion or instinct, only to some weird sequence of amino acids. Finally, biology is destiny!

This new biological model widens the application of the materialist principle. I do not share the view that it will give us the definitive science of mind because I do not accept the proposition that particular chemical or physical events and temporally related changes in mood, affect or behavior proves a causal relationship. These are relationships but that does not eliminate others which are also non-causal, nor does it eliminate the need for dependence on a principle of integrating and holistic activity. Likewise, any relation between molecular change and mind alteration is not so determined that free will cannot overcome it. The success the addictive personality meets with control of what is now argued to be a chemical proclivity is still an outcome dependent upon a moral choice. Biochemical defects may be part of addiction, or antisocial behavior, or any other manifestations of a disordered psyche but these do not render a person morally impotent, he can still overcome his biology. Nor is this to say that the mind is totally independent of matter, that is not the case either. Physics and chemistry (the modern neurobiology) form a basis for the possibility of mind, but only as a condition for it and not as the explanation for its richness and profundity in the autonomous person, free even to prevail over an egregious biochemistry. There is an holistic or vital psychic force which is greater than all neurobiological events. This holistic principle of mind, which gives us the man of passion, hope, fear, love and belief cannot be explained by material principles and ultimately cannot be controlled by them. None of the material factors explain consciousness any more than individual defects in anatomy, physiology or genetics add or subtract from our concept of man. All add to the incalculable complexity of mind and body and their deep interconnectedness. The molecular descriptions of mental life only verify that in some mysterious way mind is in matter and works through it while at the same time it is not itself matter. Mind is thought rather than thing, and the entire emotional life of man issues from this spiritual dimension of the biological man. There can be no spirit-man if there is not first nature-man, clearly, but these are not two independent beings rather spirit, in thought, contemplates meaning in this unity.

The old psychoanalysis and psychiatry offer greater possibilities for healing than does this new neurobiology because they allow for a healing dialogue while recognizing that psychological dysfunctions can never be solely chemical. Psychiatry, at least Jung's analytical psychology, recognized the spiritual element in mental life. Jung realized that the spiritual is a mystery which becomes solvable through the dialectic of analysis which leads the self to realization. Not so curiously, then, Jung wrote that good analysis should begin with confession, a psychological baring of the soul to the light of moral truth. Here (but not only here) a link between psychoanalysis, the medical experience, and religion, the transcendant experience, is forged. The link is further strengthened by the analytical insights that can convey to the patient the essentially religious drama that is often playing itself out in his psyche, joining medicine and theology in their mutual quest to gain for the sick man his cure.

Freud is appropriately honored for giving analysis direction and suggesting some methods. Jung, on the other hand, has more to say to contemporary man precisely because he reads his situation more profoundly, even recognizing that illness itself, neurosis for instance, is the condition for something positive to happen, a way for the sufferer to find "a new form for his finest aspirations."[9] Freud rejected the truth of the religious impulse, for him it is only primary, it answers to the dread of existence. For Freud God thinking is the psychic effluent of a people in fear of themselves, the world and the cosmos. That is how religion, God thinking, came into being, and why it persists, "when the growing individual, finds that he is destined to remain a child forever, that he can never do without protection against strange powers, he lends those powers the features belonging to the figure of his father."[10] Note that this is the same father Freud believes we all want to wish away Oedipally. Freud goes on: "(Man) creates for himself the gods whom he dreads, and whom he nevertheless entrusts with his own protection."[11] Here I think you see the contradiciton in his theory, or else you accept it in the same condition of perplexity that Freud remarked was the argument of the Church Father (Tertullian); belief (in God) because it is absurd. Freud adds, "Am I obliged to believe every absurdity, and if not, why this particular one (religion)? There is no appeal to a court above that of reason."[12] Yet he demands in his theory of the origin of religion that we do similar violence to reason.

Freud reserved his greatest criticism for religion and he believed that once it is exposed as fraudulent the false social stability it has imposed through coercion will wither. He writes anxiously, but accurately, "if the sole reason why you must not kill your neighbor is because God has forbidden it, when you learn there is no God, you will certainly kill him."[13] Freud blamed religion for regulating the masses by untruth, but he recognized that it did regulate! He hoped that we would impound religion and seek humanist goals for their own sake.

Jung could not accept this atheism. He believed that religion was the essential movement in the human experience and though he said the same thing as Freud regarding its origins he meant something much different. "At a time when a large part of mankind is discarding Christianity, it may be worth our while to understand why it was accepted in the first place. It was accepted as a means of escape from the brutality and unconsciousness of the ancient world. As soon as we discard it, the old brutality returns in force...the beast breaks loose and a frenzy of demoralization sweeps over the civilized world,"[14] an explanation the German historian Friedrich Meinicke offered for the horrors of Nazi nihilism; when the leaders of the Blackshirts tossed out God, they threw mankind away with him!

The religious question, of course, has been problematical for psychiatry throughout the twentieth century but the theory of evolution, a dominating influence in all scientific thought in our time, has been able to dismiss religion altogether. Thus, it is hardly fortuitous that the father of psychoanalysis was greatly influenced by Darwinian evolution. Psychoanalytic theory claimed to uncover some of the mechanisms of the mind but the theory of evolution had already suggested that the origins of mind lie in our zoological heritage. The two theories were connected in another way, in so far as Freud believed that the development of the individual's psychic life paralleled the biological evolution of man. Evolution even influenced social theory early on and Karl Marx presented a rational scheme of social evolution recognizing that capitalism, preminently an arrangement for the survival of the fittest, was a necessary step on the evolutionary road to the stateless, classless, demonified world of communism.

There should be little surprise that Darwin's theory gathered adherents early. In contrast to psychoanalysis and much of psychiatry, for instance, which still remain suspect scientifically, evolution has not had to compete with other scientific theories of the origin of man, it is the only theory of human origin. Equally important, for most scientists and laymen alike, a trip to the nearest museum seems to prove the theory very nicely.

The mechanisms of evolution were first discussed in scientific form in Charles Darwin's *Origin of Species* in which he presented the notions of survival of the fittest, a term borrowed from the philosopher Herbert Spencer, and natural selection, a process producing new species and eliminating others through gradual, random and passive change.

The main elements of the theory came from several sources. Darwin's Grandfather, Erasmus Darwin, had been influenced by Adam Smith's political economy of free competition allowing the best to succeed. This was incorporated into Charles Darwin's theory of competition in nature while Thomas Malthus's, book on population and food supply greatly influenced him for there he first met the "struggle for life." Another important influence came out of the geologist Charles Lyell's work on gradual change rather than sudden (catastrophic) change in forming the earth strata. When Darwin finally penned his book this gradualism was a major part of his ideas about changes in nature. All of these came together after Darwin's trip to South America on "The Beagle," a trip which allowed him to observe the struggle for life first hand.

The voyage of the Beagle lasted close to five years and for twenty years thereafter Darwin worked assiduously on breeding experiments and statistical research to shape his theory into scientific form. Finally, in 1858, with the encouragement of scientists in England and with the impetus of similar work by Alfred Russell Wallace, Darwin read a paper before the Linnean Society in London. This led to the publication of the *Origin of Species,* in 1859, a book which was an overnight success, in good measure due to its support among Linneans. There was another reason for this success, however, Darwin's views on the processes of nature complemented growing English theories about society and economy. The upper class Englishman and the intellectual were promoting an individualistic, competitive theory of society, a survival of the fittest philosophy. The Origin of Species offered a biological "economy of nature," as it were, in line with social and economic thinking of the time. Obviously Darwin was not promoting his theory as a social theory, or even as an impediment to theology. Nonetheless, his theory became the basis for social Darwinism (let the best prevail) and, more significantly, a popular intellectual argument against Biblical revelation. Darwin, on the other hand, simply wanted to present a theory of evolution in nature hoping that the skeptics would accept fitness and selection with the understanding that these were discussed, as he said, metaphorically. "All results follow from the struggle for life. Owing to this, variations, however slight, if they be in any degree profitable to individuals will tend to their preservation and will generally be inherited. I call this principle by which each slight variation, if useful, is preserved by the term natural selection, but survival of the fittest is more accurate...I should premise that I use this term in a large and metaphorical sense."[16]

Metaphors, of course, are not scientific statements and Darwin realized that it would be difficult to convey the specific meaning of selection and fitness. In his book he stated that, "In order to make clear how, as I believe, natural selection acts, I beg permission to give one or two imaginary examples,"[17] which he did by citing the obvious, survival of the strongest among predators, and adaptation among plants. The problem, of course, is that stating the obvious is proof of nothing in the case of evolution because it does not explain how the obvious is as it is. Darwin tried to reassure us by noting that "when we reflect on the struggle we may console ourselves with the full belief that the war of nature is not incessant, that no fear is felt, that death is generally prompt and the vigorous, the healthy and the happy survive and multiply."[18] Certainly, that added nothing to the theory either but it did help convey the idea that the theory reflected the good sense and benevolence of nature.

The spread of Darwin's theory was a major intellectual event of the nineteenth century and has had profound implications right up to the present time. The great debates did not revolve around its scientific validity, however, as most everyone then conceded the point. The real issue was theological. Did Darwinian evolution remove God from the natural world? Certainly the idea of gradual processes of change in nature determining the genesis of life and regulating its diversity put the Biblical account to task. Many took it to mean that man is descendent from lower forms and is not a special creature, only first among the primates. This is a view which fit nicely with the growing materialistic, mechanistic view of human life that was issuing from the medical research laboratory in the nineteenth century. Man, the great beast, functions as an animal because he is a relative, driven, as other animals, by instinct and physiology. Darwin, himself, did not deny a role for God (he suspended judgement) but his theory was used by others to advance the idea of zoological man.

Evolution certainly was congenial to the atheism of Feuerbach and Marx, and Freud specifically credited the theory with considerable influence on his medical career and professed atheism. For many others who subscribed to the materialistic (non-spiritual) interpretation of man's existence evolution provided scientific support for their position. Evolution suggested that the world of nature moves as inexorably as the silent physical world and cosmos, following its own laws of survival, generation and extinction. Man has no special purpose in this world of nature; he is only the most adaptable and fittest of the animals. Early on, then, the theological and the scientific clashed, the theists continued to believe in special creation, and the atheists used Darwinian theory to support mechanistic biogenesis operating by its own principles without spirit or purpose. And from the beginning paleontological findings were introduced to show the links between man and ape.

Among the most recent attempts to use paleontology to bolster this view has been the research on an ape named Lucy. *Lucy, the Beginnings of Human Kind,* by Donald Johanson, was published in 1977 and was hailed as a breakthrough because it presented evidence for bipedalism (upright posture) in apes. I suppose this "evidence" was impressive precisely because it fulfilled the old dictum that "man stands alone for he alone stands." In any case, "Lucy" advanced the notion that the transition from ape to human occurred after apes achieved bipedalism, implying that food gathering changed and tool making became possible (if the front feet aren't feet then they must be hands!). Most importantly, bipedalism allowed that most human of experiences; pair bonding.

Prior to Lucy, as the story goes, apes could breed and nurture slowly because food sources were abundant. With climatic change, however, food became scarce and the ape had to reproduce more quickly or die out. But "one species hardship is another's opportunity" and Lucy and her fellows evolved a means for faster reproduction. As a result of this evolutionary pressure, "monogamous pair bonding developed and the male began helping in food gathering."[19] Lucy (to name her is to know her, like the girl next door) was a kind of protohuman, upright, ambulatory and monogamous, a four foot relative who walked several million years ago.

Paleontologists use this kind of "evidence" to strengthen their claim that continuing examination of fossil records will secure the argument for the descent of man. But no amount of fossil evidence or accumulation of Lucy-like specimens can finally validate the claim since this is evidence by enumeration. This is tenuous enough in its own right but it also assumes that the scientific methods for fossil dating and the time scale of evolution are correct. But some scientists desagree with these points. They note that evolution by enumeration escapes the need to demonstrate how the putative molecular mechanisms of evolution bring morphologic changes and speciation at the gross level. Others reject the time specificity of dating technologies and admit the possibility of periods of accelerated or "punctuated" evolution, the first hint that catastrophism may one day return to favor.

As a result of long standing debate over these aspects of the fossil record some evolutionists have shifted from fossil studies to primate studies, emphasizing psychological links between man and ape. Some biologists claim that the evidence that higher primates possess human like language and learning skills is far more persuasive than the paleontological data in marking the descent of man. Some of these "functionalists" even promote their argument by their own criticism of fossil evidence as inadequate to show evolution "at work." Others incorporate the psychological data (ape "language," "emotions" and "social life") with the fossil data to support evolutionary theory from functional and structural perspectives.

One of the best known popularizers of evolution, astrophysicist Carl Sagan, spends considerable time discussing this kind of evidence in his book *Dragons of Eden,* developing his points with more fanciful notions and metaphors than usually grace a book on science. Sagan accepts the usual descent from ape business and notes with enthusiasm that "powerful selective forces evolved organisms with grace and agility and an intuitive grasp of Newtonian gravitation. Human intelligence is fundamentally indebted to the millions of years our ancestors spent aloft in trees,"[20] and he even goes on to suggest that man's desire to fly is the result of the memory of our life in the trees. He wonders why we came out of the trees but without answering the question (He can't) adds that "after we returned to the savannah and abandoned the trees did we long for those great leaps? Is the daytime passion for flight a nostalgic reminiscence of those days gone by in the branches?"[21]

Professor Sagan discusses chimp language with the same zeal, offering it as another proof of the evolutionary connection. According to Sagan and other ape-language theorists human language skills are an extension and refinement of the same capacity in our primate forbears. In his book Sagan describes experiments in which chimps were taught American sign language, the chimps then using this to match objects with their appropriate signs. Sagan marveled at the chimp Lana who "having never seen a spherical fruit other than an apple...seeing an orange signed the word 'orange apple'...after having burned her mouth on a radish she described radishes as 'cry,' 'hurt,' 'food' in sign."[22] Sagan even expressed amazement at chimp "computer skills" and offers that "it is difficult to see any difference in quality between chimp gesteral language and ordinary speech in children."[23] Sagan even suggests an emotional "high" for the chimps who are using their new found language. He writes, "it is hard to imagine the emotional significance for chimpanzees of learning language"[24] and he compares their excitement with Helen Keller's reaction when she first communicated meaning by sign. "I felt eager to learn," Sagan quoted Keller, "everything had a name and each name gave birth to a new thought. Every object seemed to quiver with life."[25]

Scientists who work with primates have had little hesitation in molding the chimp-language evidence in the same fashion as Sagan makes use of it, exhibiting it as a "functional" missing link. There should be little surprise that chimps can communicate, all living things communicate through instinct and association. But any scientist should know that there is an absolutely qualitative and unbridgeable difference between animal communication, signing, association etc. and human language. The human skill is no single or simple skill, instead it represents the totality and complexity of man's consciousness. Other living things can communicate but only human communication can transcend the immediate and cross time. Only human language is expositional, allegorical, metaphorical and anagogical, it is no mere sign or utterance, it is the how of thinking. Logos is word and thought.

Sagan's examples of chimp language, and newer research in which chimps supposedly develop a vocabulary that they can retrieve on computers all describe a skill, no doubt, but it is a learned skill absolutely dependent on the human factor. A chimp may make a particular sign, punch out a specific word or repeat a sound that has been previously matched to the object presented to it. The chimp makes the association between sign and object but it is the passive recipient of all of the data and structure in the experiment. Men introduce the sign and conceptualize the logo. The chimp is taught to connect the two, but the chimp only connects, it does not turn to teach its mates nor does it build a structure or syntax beyond the elements presented. There is no spontaneous development of logos, the chimp neither abstracts nor conceptualizes. Conceptualization is on a far different order of things, it is on the order of things that makes our language/thought the specifically and uniquely human experience it is.

The uniqueness of human language, its singular power and depth, is revealed by watching its development in young children. Infants and toddlers move quickly from the association-signing proto-language that bears only a superficial relation to chimp language to complex patterns of human language-thought. With the acquisition of a mere few hundred words, the development of the syntactical arrangement, and the growth of conceptualization, children can build a language, any language, while they build understanding and comprehension. Here the word, ideogram, glyph, gesture, etc.

move to a higher level of human function and become a basis for the profound and diverse experiences of full human language, which makes man unique in nature,[26] the point the evolutionists try to make in using chimp language as an important proof of our descent from apes misses this difference completely. The real message from Lana and Lucy and all the other apes is simply this; real language is the discovery of meaning and meaning is our special province, man is the "meaning giving being."[27]

The interest in chimp language for evolution is essentially an extension of the idea of establishing the ape-man link by studying the behavior of apes rather than their fossil history but another area of research has shifted the emphasis from the anatomic and functional to the molecular level. The identification of the basic biochemistry of genes and the development of new technologies which can manipulate genetic material has been the basis for the molecular scientists' claim that they have solved the problems inherent in older evolutionary theory. They readily admit that selection and fitness were elusive concepts and that paleontology was not going to reveal them. They argue that the effects of molecular evolution are not to be sought in individual organisms but in populations of genetic material, large populations which successfully meet the mutation pressure of selection which produces a grand evolutionary movement through "differential reproduction." Putting it equally obliquely, fitness is conferred by higher "net production rates" having less to do with the numbers of surviving offspring and more with the chances of begetting offspring which yield offspring who survive.

Sir Peter Medawar, a Nobel winner in biology, has been a leading exponent of molecular evolution, and has loudly proclaimed molecular selection and fitness. Sir Peter notes that

> it is not the lineages of descent but whole animal populations that undergo evolution. The population that was deemed to undergo evolution could best be thought of as a population of fundamental replicating units of genes rather than a population of individual animals or cells. Natural selection can now be measured in terms of the net reproductive advantage of the replication unit. This is essentially a measure of the degree to which the unit prevails over competitors or alternatives."[28]

Medawar is really saying that the fossil record was the wrong place to look for evolution, its real locus is the genes and the mechanisms are molecular. Mutations are genetic events induced by the pressure of the environment, leading to a redistribution of gene pools through selection. One of the points of this is that corresponding changes at the gross, i.e., observable, scale are not necessarily either temporally or specifically related to these mutations.

Medawar and the molecular biologists are only shifting the emphasis without producing the explanation. They are giving us molecular "newspeak" while serving up the same old theories and mechanisms in a richer text of obfuscation. Medawar, of course, takes exception to such criticism, "in evolutionary theory there is no proof of evolution as crushingly decisive as pictures proving the earth is round. The reasons that have led professionals to accept (evolution) are in the main too subtle to be grasped by laymen."[29] Very well, but I'm waiting for the pictures.

The molecular biologists have introduced another "proof" of evolution, more a kind of comparative molecular anatomy than molecular explanations of selection and fitness. Molecular anthropologists have emphasized the molecular similarities between human proteins and those in other primates. Apes, for instance, have DNA structures which agree with ours within one to two percentage points. Other data shows that man and ape have closely related molecular sequences in enzymes, blood proteins such as albumin and the oxygen carrying protein, hemoglobin. The close relation between man and ape, then, is argued on the molecular level as well as the old gross anatomy based on the fossil evidence. The difference is that the molecular evidence is supposed to answer those objections that were continuously and validly raised about fossil proofs. In so far as the theory of evolution is explained and defined today, it is by the terms of and knowledge gained through molecular biology and, as Medawar says, remains much too subtle for the usual kind of understanding science should provide.

Any review of the highlights of evolutionary thinking, however brief, opens up the many objections to the theory, objections raised by the lack of compelling scientific explanations of the mechanisms and directions of evolution. Even the most recent discussions of evolution in terms of molecular biology fail to satisfy the demand for a clear presentation of the operations of selection and fitness. Selection may work through mutation pressure at the molecular level, well and good, but how? And what in essence is the difference between fitness conferred by virtue of the molecular arrangement and that in the real world of nature? You must recognize that in the "survival of the fittest" concept fitness occupies all the terms of the syllogism. Sure, one can say the best survive and that the best are identified by their survival but all the head scratching in the world isn't going to demystify that phrase.

There are other questions. Where are new kinds of life appearing? I don't mean animal or plant life that accomodates itself to the environ; bacteria which develop resistance to antibiotics, for instance, or aquatic life that tolerates ever increasing levels of toxins. These are adaptations, clearly, but they are not new life forms. And how about adaptation? Doesn't the term imply adaptability, and isn't adaptability a quality which inheres in living things, a quality "prior to" the environment? The answer, of course, is yes, philosophically it cannot be understood otherwise than as an inherent capacity in living things, a capacity which must mean that living things act on their environment. This can only mean that evolution is not a phenomena of the external milieu (imposed by the environment) but one of the internal milieu and one which is non-random i.e. is ordered. Thus natural selection cannot in any sense retain its original understanding with living things merely the passive recipients either of its beneficence or violence. And I don't mean that evolution is always a violent process, certainly Darwin didn't mean that even though the struggle for life impressed him greatly. No one today really holds the struggle for life idea literally. The processes of evolution are "more subtle" yet the outcome is still violent in the end, life forms either survive or wither.

This is an important point. Evolutionary theory, at bottom, is a theory about survival, the whole business of fitness, selection, adaptation is survival. On the other hand if evolution really describes the natural world then it is a world of evolutionary excess. The case of man says it all. If survival is the litmus test of evolution (I hesitate to use the word "end" as evolution rejects teleology), then primates had surged far ahead by the time of Lucy, Lucy had all the tools to get along. The appearance of man is an explosion right in the middle of a natural order ordered to survival. What place does human consciousness have in such an order if consciousness confers a radical surfeit of fitness and takes control of the whole enterprise? Human consciousness vanquishes evolution, it banishes gradualism, fitness and selection in biology because it is of a different order than biology.

Evolution through gradualism remains the scientific explanation for the appearance of man but within the scientific community there is one area of debate which poses an interesting challenge to Darwinian gradualism and is, in fact, a reformulation of the old theories of sudden, catastrophic changes that were popular before the work of Lyell and Darwin. Evolution by cataclysm (catastrophism) is a notion first advanced in this century by a psychiatrist. Immanuel Velikovsky obtained his M.D. degree from the University of Moscow in the twenties and then studied psychoanalysis under Wilhelm Stekel, a student of Freud's. Velikovsky set up an analytical practice in Haifa and Tel Aviv and developed an interest in Middle Eastern religions and mythologies. As his work progressed Velikovsky began to suspect that the Middle Eastern cosmological myths, legends and records of great natural disasters may have been telling about actual events. Velikovsky believed that catastrophism may have been an important factor in changes in nature, and one which would explain some of the inconsistencies in Darwinian gradualism. Velikovsky's evolution suggests that natural disasters, floods, fires, mammoth storms, etc. may have followed upon celestial events i.e.

comets, meteors etc., bringing a radical and sudden reordering of the ensemble of life as well as affecting the psychic experiences of peoples who lived through them. Obviously, by suggesting the psychic impact of catastrophism Velikovsky conveyed a view about the archeology of psychic life and the psychic impressions which transform mind similar to those discussed by Freud and Jung.

Velikovsky's theories have met with a good deal of ridicule from the scientific community especially as Velikovsky moves the time scale of evolution right into the middle of Pre-Christian civilizations. Today, some evolutionists are beginning to look at catastrophism, not according to Velikovsky's timetable, certainly, but with a view toward the possibility that great disasters did impose sudden and dramatic changes on an otherwise gradual and linear process.

There is another formulation of the theory of evolution which is singularly unique. It was put forth by a paleontologist, Pierre Teilhard DeChardin, who was also a Jesuit priest. It is the only formulation which deals with the radical explosion of consciousness onto the process of evolution, and it invests evolution with a profound teleology. Chardin's evolution is developed in harmony with the essential principles of Christianity. Chardin accepts the idea of evolution as a scientist but sees it as a process in the direction of spirit and God. Consciousness, in his theory, is evolving toward a state of collective perfection in a meeting with the spirit, a theological refinement of Hegel's idea of Absolute spirit and its dialectical operation in world history and a spiritualization of Bergson's *elan vital,* the impulse to life inherent in all things, a spiritual impetus to increasing harmony and perfectability. Chardin is decidedly more theological than either Hegel or Bergson, however, for him mankind is evolving in consciousness with God in a realm of collective psychism called the "noosphere." This noosphere is not part of a Platonic cosmology and Chardin's "noosphere" is not Plato's world of pure being (forms) rather it is the evolutionary movement of mankind toward the Creator. This evolution has its beginnings in the zoological, takes place in time and progresses biologically to consciousness, and finally to God-consciousness.

Chardin's is the first internally consistent Christian cosmology developed in harmony with the scientific world view of natural biological evolution. Central to Chardin's conception of the whole enterprise of "cosmogenesis" is the idea of vitalized matter which is inherently impelled toward consciousness in two directions, exteriorization (assimilation) and interiorization (psychism) in concert with a cosmos that is both evolving and involuting on itself. Chardin seems to echo Jung's theme of collective psychism which begins in the primordial archetypes of Man's prehistory. There is an important difference, however, in that for Chardin consciousness is evolving in a direction manifestly toward God in a collective movement of all psyches. Both Jung's analytical psychology and Chardin's Christianized evolution are evolutionary in so far as they draw on the archaic and accumulated collective symbolizations in the human psyche. On the other hand, Chardin's theory points to a collective psychism which is still maturing and still unfolding the meaning of existence; it is more than a collective unconscious of archaic images and archetypes.

I grant you the gross oversimplification in comparing Jung's concept of psyche with Chardin's but the point is that for both men the psyche is a spiritual place and the dynamics of psychic life are involved with spiritual symbols, meanings and needs. Chardin is a metahistorian, an evolutionist of the Divine in the world while Jung is a therapist of psychic distress as soul dysfunction but each conceives psychic life as aiming towards "integration." Chardin's theory speaks of a hyperpersonal psyche, the collective psychism of countless souls evolving spiritually. Jung's psychology is still, at bottom, an individualistic psychology of personal liberation and growth which would place the individual in harmony with himself and his fellows. Chardin lifts psychic harmony to another level, not just therapeutic harmony or integration but cosmic harmony. Chardin is not a therapist so he is not speaking the medical idiom, he is a theologian, he is speaking of the spiritual unfolding of consciousness and the meeting of man and God in psychic union through a process in time, evolution.

Chardin's theory connects to Darwin's because Chardin accepts the idea of evolution but, beyond that, Chardin is describing a spiritual movement to a specific end. In so far as Chardin's theory accepts the biological theory it, of course, suffers the same deficiencies and is no more valid a theory than Darwin's or anyone else's. One can reject all evolution theory on the strength of the argument that evolution remains a speculation based on similarities among living things and the obvious fact of change in nature. If one accepts Darwinian evolution or any of its contemporary revisions one must weigh the question of man, and the threefold question of the beginning of life, the organization of matter and the appearance of consciousness. Certainly Chardin's theory covers itself with the idea of teleological, vitalised matter but that, in fact, makes him a philosopher, not a scientist. Aside from the loftiness of Chardin's teleological evolution, he does understand the implications of consciousness for evolution. He recognizes that the human psyche takes the evolutionary process beyond the configurations of matter. Matter is now at the disposal of consciousness, and not only in the obvious way in which this is so in the everyday world but in the fundamental way that matter is extensive with consciousness, a conjunction even modern quantum theory seems to be validating. It is just not possible for matter to "complexify" or organize into a psychic power on its own, something must be infused into matter.

Consciousness, the power of intellect, the moral possibilities of free will and the certainty of existence that consciousness gives us, is the heir to all the processes of change in the physical and biological world. Unless one sees the directing hand of God touching the world and the universe, the vitalizing God who literally breathes into matter (at bottom, the Chardinian view) then the whole enterprise of evolution, as the materialists develop it, does violence to our reason. If we accept their view we are forced to say that atoms think, organized matter thinks more, and highly organized, "cerebrified," matter thinks profoundly. One would be correct to point out, however, that this means that this capacity must either be given to matter at the beginning or it is a property of matter in the sense that Aristotle's "entelechy" suggests, but either way it cannot be a property of matter sui generis!

Interestingly, the problem of matter raised by the appearance of consciousness seems to have been discovered by the scientists as well as the philosophers. It is in physics, especially quantum physics, the science of matter par excellence that the issue of consciousness-matter seems most alive. The new physics suggests that matter is not discrete or independent, quantifiable substance; consciousness must be present to "materialize" it and in doing this consciousness (the observer) imposes its own configurations on it (time, space, the relativity of matter). Classical physics rested on descriptive phenomology, the objects and motions under investigation had the same configuration, the same spatio-temporal relationships for all observers. In the new physics, the quantum world, there are only subjective realities, less "real" in the old sense and more real in subjective sense. Time, motion and mass belong to the observer and no two observers not in the same "position" know them in the same way.

Twentieth century physics has taught us that matter and energy are different aspects of the same reality, they exist together in a contradictory "structure." Matter/energy is not a constant stream of uninterrupted force but countless bundles, "quanta," of action. These quanta can exist as waves or as particles and the particular physical properties observed exist only as statistical probabilities. This indeterminateness is, in fact, a function of matter/energy in relation to the mind of the emperimenter. It is his measurement, his intervention which determines the specifics of the physical system he is examining, "man"; in the words of the Greek physicist, "is the measure of all things."

There is another point raised by the new physics. If Einstein's world view (the relative one) has replaced Newton's, it has not explained the world any better; it still has not "really" described it, other than as sets of probability equations. But physics was never simply descriptive even in its classical period. We only have to recall how the Copernican theory denied the everyday experience of all men (the sun moves, we stand still). Copernicus, however, was looking at things in a different way and was able to comprehend new relationships from old knowledge. Even Newton's gravity is illustrative of the problem. After all, universal gravity is absolutely beyond any experience of its essence; it is, in fact, a metaphysical entity. It was Newton's particular genius to "see" in commonplace events a principle, but the idea of applying this principle to all bodies everywhere was something beyond a weighing and measuring science. Newton imagined a force behind the motions of the spheres in the same way Bohr, Planck, and Heisenberg would imagine the forces of quantum activity. But quantum forces represent yet another difference in kind since this no longer imagines forces outside of the observer, but forces and properties coextensive with him.

Quantum theory is really telling us that the very basis of our knowledge in science, the principle of causality, is in question. The kind of "knowledge" physics is presenting is suggesting too many paradoxes to be resolved merely by the acquisition of new knowledge. These paradoxes question the very nature of knowledge because they do not involve the usual sets of data. As an outgrowth of this "understanding" in the new physics a number of issues now stand, some of which have important implications for the theory of evolution. Certainly, the presumption of evolution before human consciousness must be rethought based on the sense of the interwovenness of consciousness and matter that the new physics suggests. Aside from this fundamental philosophical problem (can anything exist in the absence of consciousness?) physics also has something to say about the origins of matter and life, the origin of world and cosmos which raise other paradoxes.

Let's look at one of these a bit more closely. Cosmologists have imagined that the origin of the world took place in an event called the "big bang." It is supposed that a furious explosion of ultradense matter (densely packed particles) released tremendous amounts of energy into the void (the nothing before there was something). This big bang set all of the physical processes in the cosmos and nature in motion, processes which were the impetus for the evolution of increasingly complex aggregates of matter leading gradually to human life and consciousness. The cosmologists don't say explicitly that consciousness is a derivative of the big bang, and the evolutionists do not take the big bang as the start of biogenesis. Yet, in order to reconcile the two theories we must take the whole process from big bang to Homo sapiens as a continuum, as a physico-biological unity. That, in a word, is materialism. Matter informs itself, regenerates itself and complexifies itself. Molecular biology becomes a derivative of quantum physical theory and consciousness becomes the latest (last?) arrangement of primordial matter.

There is a startling contradiction between he big bang theory, however, and another recent physical theory, the concept of "black holes." Modern cosmologists imagine black holes to be the theoretical inverse of the ultradense matter which supposedly caused the big bang. Black holes are collapsing stars which have generated such immense gravitational fields that energy is no longer able to escape. The black holes are supposedly in that state of ultradensity which presented just the right circumstances for energy to burst forth at the beginning of the universe in the first place. Yet the black holes are evidence that the universe is finite since the holes are senescent stars. The obvious question then; is ultradensity a marker for the beginning of the cosmos or a marker of a dying universe? That is what ultradensity represents in the new physics but the two expressions of ultradensity seem irreconcilable in terms of our understanding of the physical world. If ultradensity is postulated as the condition both for the birth and death of matter then the process of evolution is self-extinguishing, a positive drift (evolution) spawns its negative corollary (entropy) and that means only one thing, evolution is pointless!

Relativity theory raises its own objections as well. Relativity suggests that the energy fields in the black holes should be expanding as their matter becomes packed solid, because their mass is increasing. Yet quantum theory makes black holes collapsing energy fields because of the intensity of the gravitational fields produced by their mass. Thus ultradense matter can be understood either as the condition of tremendous implosion or else it satisfies the cosmic origin of energy and renewal, the same dilemma raised by contrasting the big bang to the black holes. There may be one escape hatch for the cosmologists, however. If the possibility of a unified field theory is real, then electromagnetic energy and gravitational fields are really "aspects" of the same physical state and the present concept of the big bang, black holes and relativity will have to be discarded since they pose a theoretical impass to a unifying theory. But the search for the conclusive evidence for the unified field has so far eluded the physicists and thus far they have been left with only the paradoxes of their science. Clearly, the paradoxes and subjectivity in the new physics raise issues that are no longer scientific but philosophical. These issues go to the very heart of the question of knowledge, surely, and not, I'm afraid, much closer to solution than when the Greeks considered them.

Biology, on the other hand, held out the longest in keeping to the requirements of the experiment in the classic sense and in holding to the idea that things exist in themselves. Biology, of course, is primarily descriptive, the experiment validates the intuition in biological research. Nonetheless, first principles in biology, as in physics, require something more than the facts. The biology experiment may describe many of the phenomena that we observe in a living system, but it is still inadequate to answer basic questions about life. You could, for instance, remove all the blood from an animal, in which case it would always succumb, but no one today suggests that the vital force or life principle resides in the blood. You cannot restore life by giving blood. The "life force" isn't in the blood. We don't know where it is. Life force, like gravity and relativity, cannot be known reductively, we can measure some of its effects and we can study life processes just as we can see the effects of gravity but we cannot see the life force any more than we can see gravity in its essence. They are, in their essence, non-demonstrable. Even if we call them "forces" carried by some physical principle we have said nothing. So we see that biology and medicine have not banished occultism. We have the same trouble with the essence of phenomena in biology and medicine as we do in physics. We only think we have certain knowledge of life because we can lay our hands on it. We can dissect, stimulate, analyze and modulate biological phenomena but we still can't scrape away enough of the old boy to find the soul, the life principle. But science is trying to settle the issue by merging biology and physics to study them with one methodology.

Biology is entering the quantum age. Many biological laws will soon be written in the same language as physical ones. The molecular level will remain useful for the study of physiological events but the quantum level is where life and matter will be joined. From a theoretical point of view the elementary particle is already regarded as the origin of all things, living and non-living. Particle physics is rewriting the bases for the theories of the ultimate composition of living matter and the whole evolutionary process. The relationship among all complex phenomena will be explained by their "ultimate" groundedness in matter and in atomism. We already have technology to see the genetic and atomic structures of living things and measure quantum lengths, smaller than four billionths of an inch. These technologies define the new medicine and they are introducing another profound change in our understanding of life. If the ancients believed life was shrouded by unseen forces our machines tell us that these forces are functions of matter and not nature mysteries, and they tell us this in the scientific way of affirmation with number and measurement.

The new concepts in science are revolutionary, no doubt, but they still leave the ultimate question unanswered; why are things the way they are? What lies behind phenomena? What is causality? What is the essence of the "forces" in cosmos and nature? Is their meaning hidden, neither ascertainable by observation or experiment, nor deducible from comprehensive physical or biological theory? It seems that all of these forces are "occult" in their essence and are metaphysical entities rather than physical ones. They are philosophical problems. When science speaks about evolution, for example, it tells us that life forms change but that whole idea presumes a principle of action within living things and within the matter from which they issue. At the same time evolution is only describing the acquisition of new traits and the results of change, not the dynamic process itself. Acquisition and change presuppose interaction between subject and environment in a way that science cannot explain. If the evolutionary movement to consciousness is a function of arrangements of matter, an arrangement which at the quantum level gives matter those occult qualities it does not possess in the world of everyday things, this movement is impossible unless we assume that matter shares in consciousness in the cosmos, and Chardin's idea of the "Cosmic Christ," the unfolding of the Divine in the world, is the only one which answers the problem. However unscientific this is as an answer, it certainly takes account of the evidence as science has given it and demands no greater metaphysical leap than any "occult-scientific" answer would demand.

The new biology of the mind, the neurobiology that is displacing analytic theory, makes the same kind of demand. Neurobiology asks us to believe that the whole (mind) is the sum of its parts (chemical and anatomic) and says that the aggregate has a non-material function, thought. Then LaMettrie, Cabanis and Karl Vogt were right: thought oozes from the brain like juices issue from organs. And science will even give you machines which confirm this by artificial intelligence, an "intelligence" of integrated circuits which mimics the mind with its neurochemical circuits. We don't yet know how we think but we claim that we have made a machine that thinks.

The point is that human consciousness is absolutely unique, it is the only indeterminate function in nature. Matter and consciousness are related only because consciousness dominates matter and all physical events in so far as it "materializes" them. If evolution was the "plan," then the projection of consciousness onto nature was the only unfinished business of evolution. Now consciousness will direct all of the phenomena in life and take part in the creative movement. There will no longer be any cosmic business that is conducted without us, no "artificial" life that does not take some element from human life, no artificial intelligence which is not based on our intelligence, no evolution that does not issue through us.

Any explanation which science may offer for the appearance and the workings of human consciousness can only be an "occult" explanation, that is an explanation which imputes spiritual (non-material) qualities to matter. This "occultism" is perhaps one of the biggest problems facing contemporary science because it places science right in the middle of what are essentially philosophical issues.

Contemporary biology and physics are forcing us into speculations which are every bit as involved in "occultism" as all that has passed before. One physicist put it that physics (and it's equally true in biology) is not in need of "precision" but "key overview ideas" and a Cambridge mathematician calls for an "intuitive leap" in describing the cosmos. What could they mean since they obviously do not mean simple reductivist science? Obviously, the cosmos obeys laws, Nature obeys laws. Nature does not present itself in chaos, nor is the cosmos flying away. Whtever has been described fits into the harmony of the whole, but then that is the necessity of the cosmos! Even the principle of indeterminateness speaks in physics to events governed by physical laws, its quibble is statistical (which manifestation of the physical law is presented to us at the particular instant we peak in?). Likewise, something as haphazard appearing as the physiology of disease reveals the same ordered behavior as the rest of matter and life. Disease may be disagreeable biology but it is hardly biology in chaos, it must follow its own "laws." Whether one starts with the broadest kinds of generalizations or begins by working up from bits and pieces, however we examine the world or nature we find them orderly. The question remains—How? Is all of this the "occult" property of matter, or has someone's hand infused order into nature and life into matter?

Science stands firm in its proposition that all is orderly in its essence. Matter has organized itself. Religion says all is ordered because God is there. If one chooses materialism and the idea that matter, of itself, authors all life and consciousness, then one must confront the oldest and thorniest of philosophical questions, how can the "life principle" inhere in matter. Those who choose a theological explanation offer that matter and life depend, ultimately, on the "First Cause."

Western science, itself, derives from the belief in the rational world of first cause. Spengler's claim that "there is no natural science without a precedent religion"[30] is a claim based on that fact. We may be able to develop a philosophy of science but there can be no valid scientific philosophy, any ultimate scientific key to the origin and meaning of the cosmos, of life, of human existence. Science might take us closer to the answer even as its advances reveal the limits of its own inquiry but questions of meaning cannot be answered by strictly positive (i.e. scientific) knowledge. Indeed, for the greater part of our Western intellectual history the answer was presumed and science, as it developed, reinforced the presumption, as our short narrative has pointed out. Questions of meaning were referred back to the theological explanation, even the idea of science itself and the exposition of the laws of nature and cosmos presupposed a theological universe. Only in our day is the theological presupposition incredible and positive knowledge put in its place. But the paradoxes of science and the insufficiency of its methods have flung open the gates and a flood of scientific explanations are offered to settle man's oldest questions. Evolution says man is an animal, psychoanalysis says he behaves like one, and physics says the animal is "living" matter. Man is the most developed product of the primordial slime that started the world. This is the point about science in the twentieth century, it is blatantly and obsessively materialistic because we have transformed its message. We have embraced positivism and emptied knowledge of all spiritual links. Both modern science and positivist philosophy have severed their previous connection with a theological universe.

The positivist spirit has taken over all contemporary thought so that all of the disciplines involved in the study of man and his culture study them scientifically, positivism is the standard. Hence all the "social sciences," social and industrial psychology, the sociology of crime, poverty, family, etc., modern historiography, economics and political theory, anthropology, even jurisprudence, have been reduced to weighing and measuring. All of them quantify human activities and study them in the same way medical researchers study man in the laboratory, as a specimen.

Medical thought has contributed to and borrowed from this positivism, and modern medical thought has been in the specific direction of scientific knowledge and away from the spiritual in man, as our review has shown. This medical positivism is a large part of the reason why medicine is ill prepared to deal with ethical, moral and practical issue on its own. I suggested earlier that medical thinking no longer thinks about the "whole man," there are only men with physical or mental defects, social inadequacies, borderline personalities, cultural maladjustment, inferior genetics, or negative life experiences. Each of these debilities requires its own specialist.

This brings us to the other problem with science, and not only medical science. Man can no longer comprehend all of the scientific statements about him. The molecular biologist and geneticist speak of theories which by their own admission are "too subtle" for him, and the physicists are presenting cosmological theories that are paradoxical, so modern man can have no real connection to the cosmos intellectually, and science will not allow him a connection that is naturalistic. If the primitive had nothing but his spiritualistic image of the heavens and nature, these, at least, made nature and cosmos relevant and gave him a sense of place in the cosmic order. Modern man, on the other hand, neither knows nor spiritualizes. His scientific "knowledge" is not the common property of men but the esoteric obscurations of professional elites. And his spiritual life... well, to the extent modern man has lost it he is just as Nietzsche said of him, "I am everything that knows not which way to turn."[31]

The present state of affairs leaves us with two questions, what knowledge can we trust is really knowledge, and does scientific knowledge leave a place for God? Certainly the new physics, more than any other science, suggests the problematical nature of knowledge, and seems to put to rest the idea that there is an objective world commonly agreed upon. Thus, in a milieu of "conditional" knowledge, thinking about knowledge, truth and being is open ended and one is free to choose his metaphysics. The acceptance of the idea of a subjective universe can only mean the end of the normative one. But if we reject the idea of a normative universe what becomes of science? Can there be a valid science of the subjective? Does this mean the withering of the new metaphysics?

Our response can only be an appeal to the common-sensical witness of experience, science itself, and the old presumptions about man and cosmos that made science thinkable in the first place. Western civilization and Western science (indeed there is no other) rest on the presumption of "reality," ours is a world of order and reason, the world is comprehensible precisely because there can be no science otherwise. Man's mastery over nature, however we take it, certainly calls for some kind of nature which is "really there."

The religious question is inextricably bound to this because it takes a basis in reason from those same presumptions. Science, of course, has come so far in its demand for objectivity that it has called into question the very possibility of "real" knowledge. Religion, on the other hand, has remained firm in holding out an objective meaning for man and his place in the cosmic order, objective in the sense that the meaning is the common possession of all men, objective in that man and cosmos issue from creation. The meaning, therefore, is theological, not rational, but that isn't to say that the meaning is irrational. The point is that the validity of scientific knowledge cannot rest on its own propositions, on any scientific or positivist theory of knowledge. All knowledge rests on some truths held a priori, beyond demonstration. When science seeks to define these and takes nothing as true or primary it is a confusion of tongues. Each generation of scientists brings its own "knowledge" and explication of the world, cosmos and man. I don't mean that the scientist should abandon this quest for knowledge, he is charged with this mission and his knowledge must be examined on its own merit, by its own propositions. But then it must be weighed in another step which is philosophically open. For that reason more than any other science and philosophy must produce a new synthesis.

A new synthesis will give man his world once again, a place in the cosmic order. In such a synthesis scientific knowledge counts because it is a way to truth. I said that science introduced a new world view by deposing belief, but that is not precisely how it happened. Knowledge and power seduced us into the belief that science would answer all of our questions with a scientific philosophy. Science did not change us so much as we changed the meaning of the message. Perhaps it is simply the case that man is no more gifted intellectually than before but has only applied his intellect to different problems, choosing to answer some questions rather than others, or to answer them all in the same way, scientifically. On the other hand, it is imperative that science maintain a rigorous standard which, in fact, has dissolved as science has claimed social theory, psychology, economics, politics and history. Here the scientist can offer no security about the validity of knowledge and should speak out against building "facts" into scientific truth in areas of human activity where the imponderable always outweighs the predictable. This is true not only for bastard science, it fits equally well those we have come to accept as legitimate, objective, valuefree; the very point about psychoanalysis, evolution and physics. Certainly any man's theory of the subconscious is as good as the next, any theory of the mind bound to be riddled with subjectivity and paradox. Likewise, the flaws in evolutionary theory and the question of the "really real" in the new physics speak to the insufficiency of purely scientific propositions about man and cosmos there are no theories of propositions which can stand outside a coherent context, and science cannot provide that alone.

Notes

Introduction

[1] Konrad Heider, *De Fuehrer,* trans. Ralph Manheim (New York: Lexington Press, 1944), p.231.
[2] G.W.F. Hegel, *On Art, Philosophy and Religion,* ed. J. Glenn Gray (New York: Harper and Row, 1920), p. 141.
[3] Ibid.
[4] C.S. Lewis, *The Abolition of Man* (New York: Macmillan, 1973), p. 69.
[5] Karl Jaspers, *Man in the Modern Age* (Garden City: Anchor Doubleday, 1973), p. 188.
[6] William Sullivan, "The New Physics," *New York Times Magazine* (March 24, 1982), p. 104.
[7] René Dubos and J.P. Escando, *Quest: Reflections on Medicine, Science and Humanity* (New York: Harcourt, Brace Jovanovich, 1979), p. 60 .

The Shaman

[1] J.J. Bachofen, *Myth, Religion and Mother Right,* Trans. Ralph Manheim, Bollingen Vol. XIV (Princeton: Princeton University Press, 1967), p. 16.
[2] Owen Barfield, *Saving the Appearance* (New York: Harcourt, Brace, Jovanovich, 1965), p. 41.
Mircia Eliade, *Myth, Dreams and Mysteries* (New York, Harper Colophon, 1975), p. 61.
[4] Ibid.

[5] Joseph Needham, *Science, Religion and Reality,* (New York: George Braziller, 1955), p. 80.

[6] Eliade, *Myth, Dreams and Mysteries,* p. 14.

The Way

[1] Charles Moore and Sarvepalli Radhakrishnan, ed. *Source Book of Indian Philosophy* (Princeton: Princeton University Press, 1957), p. 49.

[2] Ibid., p. 13.

[3] Ibid., pp. 305-306.

The Greeks

[1] Plato, *Works of Plato: The Phaedo,* Franklin Library (1979), pp. 392-393.

[2] Frederick Coppleston, *History of Philosophy* (Garden City: Doubleday Image, 1962), p. 106.

[3] Plato, *The Charmides,* pp. 6-7.

[4] Ibid., *The Phaedrus,* pp. 243-244

[5]

[6] Hippocrates, *The Writings of Hippocrates: The Epidemic,* Franklin Library (1979), p. 111.

[7] Ibid., *Ancient Medicine,* p. 10.

[8] Ibid., *On Regimen,* p. 73.

[9] Ibid., *The Epidemic,* p. 133.

[10] Aristotle, *Aristotle's Works: The Analytics,* Franklin Library (1979), p. 61.

[11] Ibid., *The Topics,* p. 227.

[12] Ibid., *The Posterior Analytics,* p. 155.

The Middle Ages

[1] Johann Huizinga, *The Waning of the Middle Ages,* (New York: Doubleday Anchor, 1954), p. 10.

[2] Hugh Pope, *Augustine of Hippo,* (Garden City, New York: Image, 1961), p. 229.

[3] Moses Maimonides, *On the Causes of Symptoms,* ed. J.O. Leibowitz and Sitlomo Marcus (Berkeley: California, 1974), p. 15.

[4] Ibn Khaldun, *The Muqaddimah: An Introduction to History,* trans. Franz Rosenthal, Bollingen XVIII (Princeton: Princeton University Press, 1967), p. 102.

[5] Christopher Dawson, *Medieval Essays* (Garden City: Image Books, 1952), pp. 121, 123.

[6] Ibid.

[7] Jolande Jacobi, ed., *Selected Writings of Paracelsus*, trans. Norman Gutterman, Bollingen XXVIII (Princeton: Princeton University Press, 1964), p. 66.

[8] Ibid., p. 38.

[9] Ibid., p. 50.

[10] Ibid., p. 55.

[11] Ibid., p. 57.

[12] Ibid., p. 72.

Early Modern Science

[1] "The Last Days of Copernicus," *The National Magazine*, July 1852.

[2] E.A. Burtt, *Metaphysical Foundations of Modern Science*, (Garden City, New York: Doubleday Anchor, 1954), p. 59.

[3] Ibid., p. 57.

[4] Stillman Drake, *Discoveries and Opinions of Galileo*, (New York: Doubleday, 1951), p. 182.

[5] Ibid., p. 183.

[6] E.A. Burtt, *The Metaphysical Foundations of Modern Science*, (New York: Doubleday, 1954).

[7] Richard Hooker, *The Laws of Ecclesiastical Polity*, (London, 1622), p.23.

[8] Ibid., p. 25.

[9] Ibid., p. 28.

[10] William Harvey, *The Circulation of the Blood*, Everyman's Library (New York: Dutton, 1963), p. 7.

[11] Robert Hinman, *Abraham Cowley's World of Order* (Cambridge: Harvard University Press, 1960), p. 18.

[12] Roger Pilkington, *Robert Boyle: The Father of Chemistry* (London: John Murray), p. 160.

[13]

[14] John Lowthorp, *Philosophical Transactions to the Year 1700*, vol. III, (London, 1749).

[15] Ibid., p. 25

[16] Ibid., p. 26.

[17] Ibid.

[18] Ibid.

[19] Ibid., p. 27.

[20] Ibid.

[21] Ibid., p. 29

[22] J. Cory Jefferson, *A Book About Doctors* (London: Hurst-Blackett, 1847), p. 60.

[23] Ibid., p. 62.

[24] Ibid., p. 63.

[25] Ibid., p. 65.

[26] Ibid., p. 66.

[27] Ibid., p. 68.

Eighteenth-Nineteenth Century

[1] Ernst Cassirer, *The Philosophy of the Enlightenment* (Princeton: Princeton University Press, 1951).

[2] Ariel Durant and Will Durant, *The Age of Voltaire*, Story of Civilization Series (Simon & Schuster).

[3] Rudolph Steiner, *The Riddles of Philosophy* (Spring Valley, New York: Anthroposophic Press, 1975), p. 221.

[4] Ibid., p. 263.

[5] Ibid., p. 267.

[6] Claude Bernard, *Introduction to Experimental Medicine* (New York: Henry Schuman, 1949), p. 185.

[7] Burtt, *Metaphysical Foundations* p. 160.

[8] Bernard, *Introduction to Experimental Medicine*, p. 160.

[9] Ibid., p. 192.

[10] Ibid., p. 184.

Twentieth Century

[1] Rudolph Steiner, *The Riddles of Philosophy* (Spring Valley, New York: Anthroposophic Press, 1973), p. 178.

[2] Adolph Grunbaum "How Valid is Psychoanalysis," *The New York Review of Books* (March 5, 1981), p. 40.

[3] F. Neitzsche, *The Gay Science*, Trans. Walter Kaufman (New York: Vintage Books, 1974), p. 288.

[4] Paul Ricoeur, *The Symbolism of Evil*, (Boston: Beacon Press, 1969), p. 15.

[5] Martin Buber, *Pointing the Way*, trans. Maurice Friedman (New York: Schocken Books, 1974).

[6] J. Kockelmas, ed., *On Heidegger and Language*, (Evanston, Illinois: Northwestern University Press, 1972), p.29.

[7] Carl Jung, *Psychological Reflections: A New Anthology of His Writings*, R.F. Hull & Joland Jacobi, eds., Bollingen, vol. 31 (Princeton: Princeton University Press), p. 84.

[8] Ibid.

⁹ Martti Siirala, *Medicine in Metamorphosis*, (London: Tavistock Publications, 1969), p. 26.

¹⁰ Jung, *Psychological Reflections,* p. 88.

¹¹ Sigmund Freud, *The Future of an Illusion,* New York: W.W. Norton and Company, 1975), p. 24.

¹² Ibid., p. 27.

¹³ Ibid., p. 28.

¹⁴ Ibid., p. 29.

¹⁵ Jung, *Psychological Reflections,* p. 344.

¹⁶ Charles Darwin, *Origin of Species,* (Franklin Library, 1979), p. 36.

¹⁷ Ibid., p. 37.

¹⁸ Ibid., p. 38.

¹⁹ Boyce Rensberger, "About to be Human," *New York Times Book Review,* (February 22, 1981), p. 61.

²⁰ Carl Sagan, *Dragons of Eden,* (New York: Random House, 1977).

²¹ Ibid., p. 91.

²² Ibid., p. 92.

²³ Blaise Pascal, *Pensees,* (New York: E.P. Dutton, 1958), p. 101.

²⁴ J. Kockelmas, *On Heidegger and Language*, p. 60.

²⁵ Jean and Peter Medawar, *The Life Science,* (New York: Harper and Row, 1977), p. 102.

²⁶ Ibid., p. 103.

²⁷ Oswald Spengler, *The Decline of the West,* Modern Library (1965), p. 104.

²⁸ Nietzsche, *The Antichrist,* (New York: Penguin Books, 1969), p. 115.

²⁹ Thomas Mann, *The Magic Mountain* (New York: Vintage Books, 1969), p. 397.

Bibliography

The East

Edgerton, Franklin. *The Beginning of Indian Philosophy.* Cambridge: Harvard University Press, 1970.

Finnegan, J. *The Archeology of World Religion.* Princeton: Princeton University Press, 1952.

Moore, Charles, and Radhakrishnan, Sarvepalli, ed. *A Source Book in Indian Philosophy.* Princeton: Princeton University Press, 1957.

Palos, Stephen. *The Chinese Art of Healing.* New York: Herder and Herder, 1971.

Rottauscher, A. Von, and Wallnöfer, H. *Chinese Folk Medicine.* Translated by Marion Palmedo. New York: Bell Publishing, 1975.

Vogel, Virgil J. *American Indian Medicine.* Norman: Oklahoma University Press, 1977.

Zivanovic, Srbolgub. *Ancient Diseases.* New York: Pica Press, 1982.

The Greeks

Aristotle. *The Analytics.* Translated by E. M. Edghill. Philadelphia: Franklin Mint Edition 1979.

Entralgo, Pedro Lain. *Mind and Body: Psychosomatic Pathology.* Translated by Curelia Espinosa. New York: P. J. Kennedy and Sons, 1956.

――*The Therapy of the Word in Classical Antiquity.* New Haven: Yale University Press, 1970.

Galenus, Claudius [Galen], Hippocrates. *Selected Works.* Translated by A.J. Brock. Philadelphia: Franklin Mint Edition, 1929.

Herman, John Randall. *Aristotle.* New York: Columbia University Press, 1960.

Lones, Thomas. *Aristotle's Researches in Natural Science.* London: West, Newman and Co., 1912.

McKeon, Richard. *Introduction to Aristotle.* New York: Modern Library, Random House, 1947.

Mourekatos, Alexander P. *The Presocratics.* Garden City, N.Y.: Anchor Books, Doubleday, 1974.

Peter, F. E. *Aristotle and the Arabs.* New York: New York University Press, 1968.

Plato. *The Works of Plato.* Translated by Benjamin Joweh. Philadelphia: Franklin Mint Edition, 1979.

Simms, Bennett, M.D. *Mind and Madness in Ancient Greece.* Ithaca: Cornell University Press, 1980.

The Middle Ages

Aquinas, Thomas. *Aquinas Reader.* Edited by Mary Clark. Garden City, N.Y.: Image Books, 1976.

Chesterton, G.K. *St. Thomas Aquinas: The Dumb Ox.* Garden City, N.Y.: Image Books, 1956.

Copleston, F.C. *Aquinas.* New York: Penguin Books, 1977.

Dawson Christopher. *The Making of Europe.* Garden City, N.Y.: Image Books, 1952

——*Medieval Essays.* Garden City, N.Y.: Image Books, 1959.

Haskins, Charles. *The Rise of the Universities.* Ithaca: Cornell University Press, 1975.

Herr, Friedrich. *The Intellectual History of Europe.* Garden City, N.Y.: Anchor Books, 1968.

Khaldun, Ibun. *The Mugaddimah: An Introduction to History.* Translated by Franz Rosenthal. Bollingen XLIII. Princeton: Princeton University Press, 1967.

Knowles, David. *The Evolution of Medieval Thought.* New York: Vintage Books, 1962.

Maimonides, Moses. *On the Causes of Symptoms.* Edited by J.O. Leibowitz and Marcus Shlomo. Berkeley: University of California Press, 1974.

Paracelsus, Philippus Aureolus. *The Hermetic and Alchemical Writings of Paracelsus.* Edited by Arthur Edward Waite. Boulder: Shambhala, 1976.

——*Selected Writings.* Edited by Jolande Jacobs. Bollingen XXVIII. Princeton: Princeton University Press, 1969.

Phillips, R.P. *Modern Thomistic Philosophy.* London: Burns, Oates, and Washbourne Ltd., 1941.

Pieper, Josef. *Guide to Thomas Aquinas.* New York: Mentor-Omega, 1962.

Pope, Hugh. *St. Augustine of Hippo.* Garden City, N.Y.: Image Books, 1961.

Trevor-Roper, Hugh. *Rise of Christian Europe.* New York: Harcourt, Brace and World, 1967.

Weisheipl, James. *The Development of Physical Theory in the Middle Ages.* New York: Sheed and Ward, 1959.

Early Modern Science

Boas, Marie. *The Scientific Renaissance*. New York: Harper and Row, 1966.

Burtt, E.A. *Metaphysical Foundations of Modern Science*. Garden City, N.Y.: Anchor Books, 1954.

Cassirer, Ernst. *An Essay on Man*. New Haven: Yale University Press, 1974.

——*The Individual and the Cosmos in Renaissance Philosophy*. New York: Harper and Row, 1964.

Drake, Stillman. *The Discoveries and Opinions of Galileo*. pp. 182-189. New York: Doubleday, 1957.

Hinman, Robert. *Abraham Cowley's World of Order*. Cambridge: Harvard University Press, 1960.

Hooker, Richard. *Of the Laws of Ecclesiastical Politie*. pp.15-18. London, 1622.

Lowthorp, John. *Philosophical Transactions to the Year 1700*. vol. III. London, 1749.

Nicolson, Marjorie Hope, *Pepy's Diary and the New Science*. Charlottesville: University of Virginia Press, 1960.

Westfall, Richard. *Science and Religion in Seventeenth Century England*. Ann Arbor: University of Michigan Press, 1973.

Eighteenth-Nineteenth Century

Bernard, Claude. *Introduction to the Study of Experimental Medicine*. p. 164. New York: Henry Schuman, 1949.

Cassirer, Ernst. *The Philosophy of the Enlightenment*. Princeton: Princeton University Press, 1951.

Charlekors, Alan. *D'Holbachs Coterie*. Princeton: Princeton University Press, 1976.

Durant, Will and Ariel. *The Age of Voltaire*. New York: Simon and Schuster, 1965.

Gay, Peter. *The Enlightenment: An Interpretation*. New York: Vintage, 1965.

Steiner, Rudolph. *The Riddles of Philosophy*. Spring Valley, N.Y.: Anthroposophic Press, 1973.

Twentieth Century

Brown, Norman O. *Life Against Death*. New York: Vintage Books, Random House, 1977.

Buber, Martin. *Pointing the Way*. Translated by Maurie Friedman. New York: Schocken Books, 1974.

Cole, J. Preston. *The Problematic Self in Freud and Kierkegaard*. New Haven: Yale University Press, 1971.

DeChardin, P. Teilhard. *Christianity and Evolution*. New York: Harcourt, Brace, Jovanovich, 1973.

——*Man's Place in Nature.* New York: Harper and Row/Harper Colophon, 1973.

Entralgo, Pedro L. *The Therapy of the Word in Classical Antiquity.* Edited and Translated by L.J. Rather and J.M. Sharp. New Haven: Yale University Press, 1970.

Fordham, Frieda. *An Introduction to Jung's Psychology.* Middlesex, England: Penguin Books, 1973.

Foucoult, M. *The Birth of the Clinic.* New York: Vintage Books, 1975.

Frankl, Viktor. *The Doctor and the Soul.* New York: Vintage Books, 1973.

Freud, Sigmund. *The Future of an Illusion.* New York: W.W. Norton and Co., 1975.

Fromm, Erik. *The Crisis in Psychoanalysis.* Greenwich, Connecticut: Fawcett Books, 1970.

Heidegger, Martin. *Poetry, Language and Thought.* New York: Harper and Row, Colophon, 1975.

Jaspers, Karl. *Man in the Modern Age.* Garden City, N.Y.: Doubleday, Anchor Books, 1954.

Jones, Ernest. *Life and Works of Sigmund Freud.* New York: Basic Books, 1961.

Jung, Carl. *Psychological Reflections: A New Anthology of His Writings.* Edited by R.F. Hull & Joland Jacobi. Bollingen, vol. 31. Princeton: Princeton University Press, 1961

Kockelmas, Joseph J., ed. *On Heidegger and Language.* Evanston, Illinois: Northwestern University Press, 1972.

Küng, Hans. *Freud and the Problem of God.* New York: Doubleday, 1979.

Lauzan, Gerard. *Sigmund Freud: The Man and His Theories.* Greenwich, Connecticut: Fawcett Books, 1962.

Marcuse, Herbert. *Eros and Civilization.* New York: Vintage Books, Random House, 1966.

Ricoeur, Paul. *The Symbolism of Evil.* Boston: Beacon Press, 1969.

Rieff, Philip. *The Triumph of the Therapeutic.* New York: Harper and Row, 1968.

Sagan, Carl. *Dragons of Eden.* New York: Random House, 1977.

Siirala, Martti. *Medicine in Metamorphosis.* London: Tavistock Publications, 1969.

Stern, Karl. *The Third Revolution.* Garden City, N.Y.: Image Books, 1961.

General

Ackerknecht, Erwin. *A Short History of Medicine.* Baltimore: Johns Hopkins University Press, 1982.

Brick, Albert, M.D. *The Dawn of Modern Medicine.* New Haven: Yale University Press, 1920.

Castiglioni, Arturo. *A History of Medicine.* New York: Alfred Knopf, 1941.

Copleston, Fred, S.J. *History of Philosophy.* Garden City, N.Y.: Doubleday Image, 1962.

Dampier, W.C. *A History of Science*. Cambridge, England: Cambridge University Press, 1971.

Davis, Nathaniel, M.D. *History of Medicine*. Chicago: Cleveland Press, 1903.

Dunglison, Robley, M.D. *History of Medicine*. Philadelphia: Lindsay and Blakiston, 1872.

Entralgo, Pedro Lain. *Mind and Body: Psychosomatic Pathology*. Translated by Curelia Espinosa. New York: P.J. Kennedy and Sons, 1956.

Gordon, Benjamin Lee. *The Romance of Medicine*. Philadelphia: F.A. Davis, 1944.

Haggard, Howard, M.D. *Devils, Drugs and Doctors*. New York: Blue Ribbon Books, 1929.

Jaki, Stanley L. *The Road of Science and the Ways to God*. Chicago: University of Chicago Press, 1978.

Jeans, Sir James. *Physics and Philosophy*. New York: Dover Publications, 1961.

Langer, Suzanne K. *Philosophy in a New Key*. Cambridge, Mass.: Harvard University Press, 1974.

Majno, Guido. *The Healing Hand*. Cambridge, Mass.: Harvard University Press, 1975.

Massengill, Samuel Evans, M.D. *A Sketch of Medicine and Pharmacy*. S.A. Massengill Company, 1942.

Mendelsohn, Eric. *Heat and Life*. Cambridge, Mass.: Harvard University Press, 1964.

Moreno, Antonio. *Jung, Gods and Modern Man*. Notre Dame: University of Notre Dame Press, 1970

Needham, Joseph, ed. *Science, Religion and Reality*. New York: George Braziller, 1955.

Ouspensky, P.D. *A New Model of the Universe*. New York: Vintage Books, Random House, 1971.

Russell, B. *A History of Western Philosophy*. New York: Simon and Schuster, 1945.

Sciacca, Michele F. *Philosophical Trends in the Contemporary World*. Translated by Attilio Salerno. Notre Dame, 1964.

Spengler, Oswald. *The Decline of the West*. New York: Modern Library, Random House, 1965.

Steiner, Rudolph. *The Riddles of Philosophy*. Spring Valley, N.Y.: Anthroposophic Press, 1973.

Thorndike, Lynn. *The History of Magic and Experimental Science*. Vol. 8. New York: Columbia University Press, 1958.

Turner, William. *History of Philosophy*. Boston: Ginn and Company, 1903.

Walker, Richard. *Memoirs of Medicine*. London, 1799.

Weizsäcker, Carl Friedrich von. *The Unity of Nature*. New York: Farrar, Straus, Giroux, 1980.

Index